CHANG...

YOUR GUIDE TO A SLIMMER, STRONGER BODY

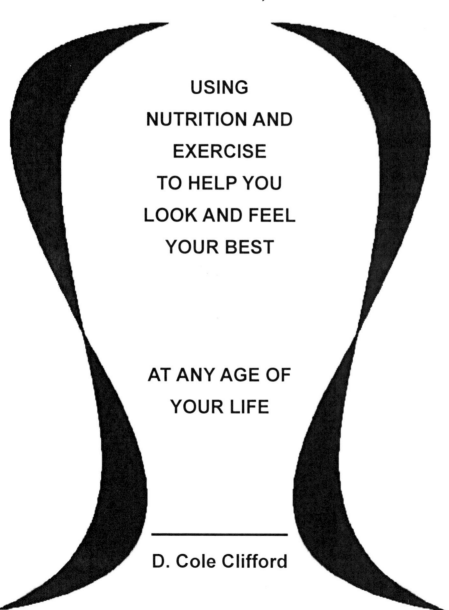

USING

NUTRITION AND

EXERCISE

TO HELP YOU

LOOK AND FEEL

YOUR BEST

AT ANY AGE OF

YOUR LIFE

D. Cole Clifford

Copyright © 2012 by D. Cole Clifford.

Library of Congress Control Number:		2012914792
ISBN:	Hardcover	978-1-4797-0048-6
	Softcover	978-1-4797-0047-9
	Ebook	978-1-4797-0049-3

All rights reserved. No part of this book may be reproduced or transmitted in any form or by any means, electronic or mechanical, including photocopying, recording, or by any information storage and retrieval system, without permission in writing from the copyright owner.

This book was printed in the United States of America.

To order additional copies of this book, contact:
Xlibris Corporation
1-888-795-4274
www.Xlibris.com
Orders@Xlibris.com
110278

CHANGING YOU

Your Guide To A Slimmer, Stronger Body

For Ashley,
Best Wishes in all
you do! / Cole

OCT. 8/15

Special Thanks to: ACI Computer Service (Burns Lake, BC)
Michael Jacques for transferal to digital format
Bonnie Jacques for final digital editing

NOTICE: All material contained in this book is for informational purposes only, and is NOT to be considered medical advice. Specific use of this information by anyone is the responsibility of that individual. Consult your physician first, if you have any pre-existing health issues that you feel might be compromised by a "proper" diet and exercise regimen, or if you believe that he or she knows more than world champion bodybuilders do, about proper health-building eating habits (nutrition), supplementation and training programs.

About the author – Cole Clifford of Burns Lake, BC

By the age of 30 Ontario-born Clifford had accumulated degrees in mathematics and education, taught high school for two years, been part of a Canadian Champion "Heavyweight 8" rowing crew for the city of Hamilton and coached two high school Canadian champion crews of his own. Moving to BC led to work in mining and logging and extensive travelling throughout the world between seasons. In 1989 he opened a gymnasium in Burns Lake, when the original version of this book was written to help his customers with the nutritional side of shaping up.

Over the course of the intervening two decades, he and his wife have continued exercising with weights 3 times per week alternating with aerobic activity, and have run a home business selling weight loss products, and continue to use them as part of a very active lifestyle. His ongoing commitment to learning about nutritional science coupled with a strong desire to help people have a healthy and active, middle and old age is what has encouraged him to add to, and to revise the original text. At the age of 63 he has just returned from competing in the British Masters rowing regatta in England, where his crew finished second overall, in the 50-55 age category.

He challenges his readers to not only embrace a lifestyle of activity supported by sound nutritional principles, but to teach it to their children and grandchildren. It's too late NOT to start, he says.

TABLE OF CONTENTS

FOREWORD

Please treat this as a reference book. This means a book that you keep on a handy shelf because you REFER to it a lot. Your goal of a changed physique is going to take quite a bit of "tunnel-vision", and it is very important that you stay centered on the ideas that will ensure your achievement. **Whatever your goal may be, you CAN achieve it within one year.** It will be difficult at times to stay "on track". You will have to remain confidently focused on the belief that your ongoing health (for the rest of your life) is worth dedicating a few hours per week to, for a year. At that point, you will have totally embraced the fitness lifestyle, and won't want to ever return to former habits. Reread these chapters many times over the next few months. You can email me personally about any concepts that are proving troublesome.

The original text of this book was written in 1990, while I was running a small gymnasium in Burns Lake, B.C. As the only employee, I spent a great deal of time going over the same information with many customers, regarding nutrition and weight loss, and it seemed easier to pull it all together in a short book and let them read it at their own pace and on their own time. I'm no scientist or researcher myself, but I have studied these topics in depth, have had some great teachers, and have asked their permission where possible, to quote from their seminar materials. In other cases, I truthfully cannot remember the names of my sources, but have full confidence in the information. It is all pretty much "public domain" stuff, some of which came verbatim from their muscle magazine articles or books. After 2 years, I had to close the doors for cash flow reasons. Although many people like to train in a gym, unfortunately very few do it all year round, and if all one's "winter customers" stop in May for a few months to go fishing and play softball, it's rather hard to survive, especially in a small town.

The original book was written in a working gymnasium and for a clientele that needed to know "the basics" of nutrition. The exercises and routines I could set up, teach, and monitor; I saw that as my job, in exchange for monthly membership dues. But the nutritional aspects of training have to be studied personally, and that is why I wrote the book. That is also why in many places throughout the book, the name of my gym, "The Change Room", is still mentioned. I left those references in for personal nostalgia's sake. Please indulge me for that. I have also left in quite a bit of text that assumed that my reader might actually wish to <u>become</u> a bodybuilder. At that time, I was not only training regular patrons who "just wanted to tone up a bit", but also providing information and guidance for those who were quite serious about body building as a sport – that is why, while some of this material is relatively simple, a lot of it is quite in-depth. Please take what you need at present, and if some of the information seems too much for you to embrace, just skip by it, and start another sub-section or chapter. I have tried to start with the simplest explanations, and work to the more complex, for those who wish or need it.

Also because of this, you may find references to the same topic referred to in different areas of the book. This is because these topics don't exist in isolation, but can be looked at from different perspectives, and I hope that any repetition you may find will at least be explained in a different way, so as to emphasize the point in question.

Some of the technical information that appears in chart (or text) form may differ from other books you may have, but not by much I imagine. There is so much research "out there", done under so many different conditions, that it would be hard to say that ANY of the numbers were "written in stone". For instance, if I state that a raw egg contains 7 usable grams of protein, and you have a book that says 6 – well, how big was the egg? We can't allow ourselves to get hung up on trivia like that. The broad strokes will do!!

Twenty years have passed since my book was first printed, and of course, there have been huge changes in our world, but not any that I know of, so far as the nutrition and exercise required for physique management goes. Building muscle size, strength and tone, and nutrition for weight <u>normalization</u> (both for those who wish to gain, as well as for those who wish to lose) still seems to be an elusive goal for many.

Over the course of the intervening two decades, my wife and I have continued exercising with weights 3 times per week, and have maintained a constant interest in the media which promotes "all the latest information". For 17 of these years, we have run a home business selling weight loss products and supplements, and continue to use them as part of a very active lifestyle. I'm not promoting those products here, but we have learned so much more than we knew back in 1990, through our involvement with the company that produces the products we market. Our ongoing commitment to learning about nutritional science coupled with a strong desire to help people have a healthy, and active, middle and old age is what has encouraged me to add to, and to revise this book. The nutritional advice given is perfect for your children as well, and your activities will be a wonderful role model for them to mimic and embrace.

I truly hope you will give this information enough serious thought to actually put it into practice, for it will certainly change the rest of your life if you do!!

The book is called "Changing You", and my gym was called "The Change Room". Funny thing is, we didn't even have one.

INTRODUCTION

You want muscles!

Yes, this statement is as true for the teenaged boy whose self-confidence needs a boost, as it is for adults **of all ages** who have let themselves get totally <u>out of shape.</u> Muscles are what give the body <u>shape</u> – whether they are huge, defined muscles like those on competition bodybuilders, or the lithe cat-like muscles on a ballerina. One thing is undeniable: MUSCLE has shape and FAT is shapeless. Fat is only metabolized (burned off) within muscle cells, so if you don't have much muscle tissue, your attempts to lose fat will be impeded. You need to build up and strengthen your muscles to enable the most efficient amount of fat loss, and THEY need to be properly fed and exercised in order to grow. That's what this book is all about.

There are many incredibly strong men and women amongst your friends, but you would never know it to look at them, because the fat layer just beneath their skin totally obscures the "definition" of their muscles. They may still look **"out of shape"**. So just <u>having</u> muscles isn't your complete desire. To look **"in shape"** your muscles need to be <u>visible</u>. That's what bodybuilding is all about.

You are interested in losing fat or gaining muscle (or both), or you wouldn't have picked this book up. Chances are that at one time or another, you have also picked up a muscle magazine like "<u>Muscle and Fitness</u>". Don't let the awesome appearance of the men and women in these magazines throw you off. It's a fair bet that their level of development is far beyond your desire, but one thing is for sure – they certainly know a lot about fat loss and muscular development, and you can learn a great deal about proper health-building nutrition and exercise performance from the articles they write.

The workout programs that I proposed at The Change Room would not turn you into a competition bodybuilder (although they were a good starting point if that was your goal), but instead utilized the time-tested principles used by bodybuilders, to help you sculpt your body into its most healthy form.

Each person's physique has genetically-controlled limitations. You cannot build huge defined arms on a marathon runner's bone structure; neither can you give a wide-hipped, narrow–shouldered physique the massive ruggedness of a Schwarzenegger. You can, however, through nutrition and training, maximize the development of what God has given you (through your ancestral background), but it must be done with respect to your individual skeletal and genetic potential.

I do not believe in attempting to become so muscular that an individual is unable to walk, or move, with ease and grace. Although such a goal would be difficult to achieve, there are some trainers in every gym who are sometimes referred to as being "muscle-bound". They walk with a strange gait, stiffly, with their arms held out widely to the sides. They have worked some muscle groups too hard or too often without regard for achieving an aesthetic appearance or flexibility. Some people I've met say that they are nervous about beginning a program of progressive-resistance weight training for fear that they will grow too big, too fast! In fact, muscles grow <u>relatively slowly</u>, (nauseatingly slowly for most of us), so you can constantly monitor and control your development very easily.

Once you start the process, you are then a <u>novice</u> bodybuilder, even if you have NO competitive desires, and this book is aimed squarely at you. As a bodybuilder, you <u>may</u> come to see your body as a "work of art". Did you smile at that one? If others can do it, why not you? You can use diet and exercise as tools, the way a sculptor uses a hammer and chisel, to create your ideal physique, the one you see in your mind's eye. Some "authorities" believe that the purpose of bodybuilding for men and women is to strive <u>solely</u> for added muscle size, but since when was a work of art judged merely by its hugeness? No – you will build your slimmer, stronger body by adding a little muscle "here and there" and subtracting a little fat "all over". It's an exciting project to undertake – this changing of your physique. It will challenge your ability to stay focused on the goal, but the ever-more-visible rewards for your efforts will far outweigh any preconceived objections you may have.

You will not be asked to spend many hours in the gym. At the beginning, one hour three times per week will suffice, as you learn the exercises, and as your body gets used to the idea that you will be imposing gradual, yet ever-increasing, demands on it. Through determination, you will encourage your muscles to "adapt" to the heavier weights being handled. They, in turn, will grow stronger, larger, and more visible, as you decrease your fat percentage through proper eating habits. This process can be begun at home with a small weight set, but a much better plan is to join a gym, get some basic information about how to do the exercises properly from the manager, and then keep learning from other members. I will outline some basic routines in Chapter 11.

If you find that you truly enjoy your workouts as a sport (sometimes referred to as "being bitten by the iron bug"), then after a few months, you will progress to a "split" system of training. You will train 4 days per week, for up to one and a half hours per session. Of course, you may <u>want</u> to train <u>more</u>, just because you love it; well, why not? as long as you aren't sustaining injuries. Your training sessions, the improvement in your health and posture, and the wonderful development you can achieve can become a very "addictive" pastime. Serious trainers almost experience "withdrawal" symptoms when forced to miss training sessions. I know I do!

In Chapter 10, I will outline the general principles of exercise that were taught at The Change Room. As mentioned previously, these methods have been developed over the last sixty years by top-flight "super achiever" bodybuilders; and the fact that they work is undeniable! I have no qualms whatsoever about presenting and teaching their methods.

The actual exercises themselves will be taught in the gym. There is no better way to learn, than through "hands-on" demonstrations. If you have several gyms to choose from, talk to each owner or manager before deciding on one. See which ones are passionate enough about their business to give you personalized, competent, on-going instruction and encouragement to achieve <u>your</u> goals. Some gyms will provide this free, while others will charge separately for it. The only thing I suggest you take is willpower – <u>lots of it</u>, depending on how much you wish to change. Ultimately your progress depends totally on <u>you,</u> and your adherence to the principles contained in this book.

It has been said that **bodybuilding is 50% nutrition**. This is because the actual "training", the performance of lifting weights for many "sets" of "reps" (repetitions), is NOT a particularly calorie-burning activity. It makes the muscles stronger and larger, but if they don't show because they are covered by a thick fat layer, the work done and time spent is largely for naught. You want <u>visible</u>, measurable results (CHANGE!).

Here's how. I do not recommend certain diets for certain people. **DIETS DON'T WORK.** Severe dieting can slow the metabolism by up to 45%. This is one reason why fat people often eat less than thin people. Another reason is that muscle *at rest* uses more energy than fat (which is always at rest). I <u>do</u> present in this book, those principles that constitute proper bodybuilding nutrition. In these few short pages is an incredible amount of valuable information – that, if applied, <u>will change</u> your body. This book contains your key to a healthier, happier life, and this I guarantee.

I give <u>you</u> some responsibility, too. I expect you to experiment, analyze, question, and think for yourself, because every "body" is different. These pages will give you your best possible launching point to control the future of your health and physique.

When Will I See Results?

If you are starting out with a "soft" body, one that is perhaps oversized around the stomach area, less than ideally formed around the thighs, and maybe a little too large around the hips and buttocks area, it will take quite an effort to get a leaner, admirable body. Slow and steady dedication will change your physique incredibly <u>over one year</u>—aren't you worth it? Of course you are. Gumption and willpower <u>will be required</u>.

Some of my (usually younger) male customers tell me at the outset that they desperately want to gain 20 or 30 pounds of muscle. They have some kind of mental image of going from a fairly gangly 150 pounds to a hulking linebacker sort of physique in a few months. Inwardly I smile, and try to think of some encouraging way to help them "dial back" their expectations to a reasonable level. I tell them to imagine the size of a one pound T-bone steak, about ¾ of an inch thick. It's big, bigger than one's hand. Since lean beef IS muscle, that size is about what a pound of muscle will look like on one's body. Now I tell them to imagine about 10 of these steaks, and to insert them on their mental image of their own body – one on each shoulder, each arm, chest and back (2 each?), each thigh, and then smooth it all out and cover it with skin. They quickly "get" the idea that a **10** pound increase in muscular weight would be pretty awesome, and acceptable, as the result of a year's steady training with good nutrition.

If you set the bar too high at the beginning, you will soon get discouraged, but if you set reasonable, achievable goals for yourself, the sky's the limit as you reset them over and over, every few months. For this reason, you will need to "pencil in" your training times amongst your other daily activities, and workouts will have to become as normal to you as brushing your teeth. It takes dedication. Think of your gym time and activities as a hobby – something that you look forward to, not as something that you HAVE to do. Your attitude has such a profound influence on what you will or will not do. You GET to go to the gym three times per week, and be around people who share your goal of physical change. Something else (like watching hours of TV), may have to take a back seat to your new habits. People who join a gym for 3 months and quit, **never** achieve their goals. You DO want CHANGE, right?

After a week, you may feel a little tauter and stronger, but no visible results are apparent. You are going to have to be determined and keep going into the gym every other day. In a few weeks, there will be a "pump", making the muscles seem larger (and they are – you can measure it!), but the pump will last only a few hours after a workout, when the muscles will return to their normal size. In a month or two, you will see some muscular development and some reduction in body fat, if you are following our nutritional suggestions as well.

People who have gotten overweight over a long period of time quite often become "used to it", even if they don't particularly like it. They actually have developed some muscles that others have not, just to transport themselves around. No matter what size you are at present, if I were to ask you to wear a backpack around everywhere for the next two weeks, filled with 50 pounds of potatoes, you probably wouldn't look forward to the prospect. It would be VERY tiring, hard on your hip, knee and ankle joints, and I'm pretty sure you wouldn't want to go for any EXTRA walking at the end of the day, never mind a few sets of tennis! Well, whether you are 10, 25 or 125 pounds overweight, getting rid of it will be like taking off that backpack. You will have more energy, less aches and pains, fit into airline seats better, maybe even play a little tennis. Now, back to the "when will I see results" question.

Fat loss (not water weight or muscle loss) at rates greater than two pounds per week, is not recommended. If you are extremely overweight, you will have to wait longer to <u>see</u> the muscles – perhaps a few months. The muscles are growing, but they are hidden under that cushion of fat beneath your skin.

In 3-6 months, specific muscles show a definite change. The pectorals (chest muscles) start to "emerge" and become well-rounded, the deltoids (shoulders) begin to show some definition (little striations show when you flex), and the entire body feels tighter and stronger.

Within six months, all muscle groups will show visible development. A cleavage line is seen in the chest (on both men and women), the delts (short for deltoids) continue to develop shape, and the thighs begin to tighten up and to show a trace of definition between the various muscles comprising the hamstrings (the back of your thighs) and the quads or quadriceps (the front of your thighs). The lats (gym talk for the latissimus dorsi, or side back muscles) may show some growth already but other small muscles can definitely be seen in your back. The most noticeable growth is in your arms. Your biceps are a little larger, and you can actually "make a muscle". On the back of the arms, your triceps begin to tighten, and <u>to show</u>, when you straighten your arm out. Nice.

In six to nine months, friends will begin to notice the changes (even when you are fully-clothed). You will begin to walk with a more athletic stride and better posture – head held high, arms not hanging down lethargically, but swinging from strong erect shoulders. By now, the lats have begun to widen, starting to give you the broad-shouldered, narrow-waisted "V" shape of an athlete, as opposed to the pear-shaped, sagging body of a sedentary man or woman.

In a year, if you are extremely diligent and pay constant attention to your training, diet, and *recuperation* (more on this when we discuss "overtraining" in Chapter 10), a perfectly symmetrical body can be yours. Even if you started out 100 pounds over-fat, it will be gone if you've constantly lost 2 pounds per week (52 weeks X 2 =104), the recommended rate. You may have some minor areas that you are still giving extra attention for greater results, but all excess body fat will be gone. Each body part will be clearly defined. People will see your biceps, triceps, chest, shoulders, back, thighs, calves, and abdominals (but only if you want them to!).

Sound good?

Study this book, and then start applying yourself.

You will never regret beginning the process, regardless of your age.

CHAPTER 1 Fat - The Enemy of Self-Esteem

The waistline is the truest indicator of your body's overall condition. If it is tight, well-muscled, and devoid of fat, then so is the rest of your body.

When a competition bodybuilder is "in shape" and you ask him or her about their condition, you won't see a flexed bicep for the proof. Instead, the bodybuilder will pull up his or her shirt and you'll be treated to a glimpse of finely sculpted, "washboard" abdominal muscles, the highly prized "6-pack"! That's the <u>real</u> test. Why? Because abs (abdominal muscles), like any muscle group, only show when the overlying adipose tissue (FAT) disappears, through proper nutrition and exercise. It is quite possible to have defined thighs, deltoids, and triceps, and still have a soft looking, smooth (or round) waistline. This is because, in general, fat gain and loss follows this rule:

FIRST ON – LAST OFF

For men, fat will be deposited on a thin, inactive body in (roughly) the following order, by body parts:

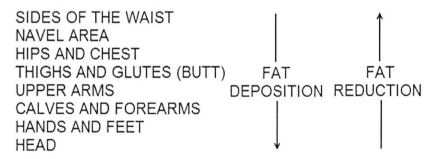

```
SIDES OF THE WAIST
NAVEL AREA
HIPS AND CHEST
THIGHS AND GLUTES (BUTT)      FAT           FAT
UPPER ARMS               DEPOSITION   REDUCTION
CALVES AND FOREARMS
HANDS AND FEET
HEAD
```

Following the "first on – last off" rule, a flat, hard midsection will become apparent ONLY after the fat stores on the rest of the body have been eliminated – through proper nutrition and a progressive, <u>consistent</u> exercise program. There is no other way, no such thing as spot reduction, and no magical shortcut.

For women, the order of body parts changes a little, since they (genetically) tend to store fat in different areas. The "trouble spots" seem to be (in general) the hips, thighs and triceps. Their body part list would look like this:

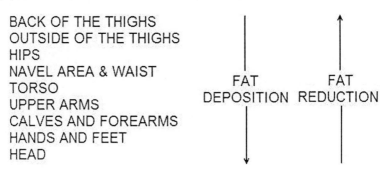

BACK OF THE THIGHS
OUTSIDE OF THE THIGHS
HIPS
NAVEL AREA & WAIST
TORSO
UPPER ARMS
CALVES AND FOREARMS
HANDS AND FEET
HEAD

FAT   FAT
DEPOSITION REDUCTION

Just as a muscular midsection is the true barometer of low overall fat level on athletes of either sex, you can be sure that a fully-clothed person with fat jowls, cheeks and chin is obese all over. Fortunately, these areas that constantly "show" lose the fat **first** when fat reduction begins.

How long does it take to get a fat-free, well-muscled midsection? That depends on you. Half of your SUCCESS depends on your persistence. The other half depends on how far out of shape you have allowed your waistline (and body) to become!

Some people can lose 10 or 15 pounds in one week, but still never succeed in attaining their goal of a slim body. Their crazy methods of diet and exercise leave them exhausted and (almost) sick, and they can't carry on with their methods (perhaps fortunately – for their overall health) to the hoped-for conclusion. Invariably, they quit the fad diet, and return to the eating habits they've always followed; then they gain back all their excess pounds, and more. There is a difference, and a vast one, between "dieting" per se, and following a sensible life-long nutritional regimen. From here on in this book, diet will mean a lifestyle habit of proper, healthy eating, not one of the current, short-term, "quick-fix" plans.

Most people think that what they have eaten all their lives is healthy, normal, and "good for them", merely because they are not currently ill. If this is true, then why are they from 10 to 100 pounds <u>over</u> the weight Nature intended? Our bodies should be lean, agile, flexible, and strong. But are they?

If you **know** that you are overweight, then you HAVE BEEN eating <u>too much</u> of the <u>wrong foods</u>. This may be the toughest fact that you will have to internalize. In all likelihood, some of the foods you have been eating contribute calories (which you need) to your body, but NO nutrients. These foods MUST be eliminated from your shelves, refrigerator, and shopping lists, as well as from your plate. Everything you eat must contribute to your goal of a slimmer body, and if some of your favorite things are detrimental to your goal, you owe it to yourself to cut them from your diet, probably <u>forever</u> – not just for a few weeks of so-called "dieting".

There have been literally thousands of books written on the subject of losing weight, yet ironically it always comes down to EATING LESS.

Less of the fat-building foods.
Less in general.

Don't waste time counting calories and working with <u>any</u> of the popular "diets" to lose weight. Obviously, larger people need more food (nutrients) to sustain their mass than those who are smaller, so we will cover what constitutes the "right amount" for YOU in a later chapter. For now, eat a little less than you are used to eating, at every meal. While it's true that natural foods are preferable (if food contains natural fiber, it moves through the system more efficiently), you can even get fat on high-fiber foods if you eat <u>too much</u> of them.

Another misconception is that you don't need willpower. **Nonsense** – it's absolutely necessary! If you don't have it naturally, drum it up. You cannot buy willpower, and you don't GET IT from your parents or your friends. How badly do you want this slimmer active physique? Tell yourself over and over that you are tired of being overweight and lethargic, that you WILL have a more muscular, dynamic body. You CAN do it! Every time you start to feel discouraged and want to slack off or quit, take yourself out behind the garage and beat yourself up. Then come back with a <u>proper</u> attitude, one which says that your goals of good health and physique are valuable, worthy of pursuit, and attainable.

Set yourself a goal and let nothing stand in your way. Don't wait for tomorrow – start right NOW. EAT A LITTLE LESS at your next meal and keep it going. If it was actually just as simple as that, I could stop typing right now. This is just the beginning – one of the first principles that you must tattoo in your mind. Eat a little less than usual.

A sensible diet coupled with an invigorating exercise plan for the whole body is the quickest, healthiest way to a well-tapered midsection, and a slimmer, stronger physique.

CHAPTER 2 Understanding Food Basics

As mentioned previously, most people believe that what they've been eating on a regular basis for years constitutes healthy nutrition. You can ask them. They assume that what "tastes good" is what the body needs. While most NUTRITIOUS foods (those that contain nutrients) taste great, unfortunately many non-nutritious foods do also! It is necessary to educate yourself as to which foods contain the nutrients you need, which ones do not, and then eliminate the foods which do not contribute to your goal of a slimmer, stronger body.

It is possible to eat **lots** of delicious, nutritious food and not get fat. There is no reason ever to be hungry when healthful eating habits are established. Forget "diets" and the years of seemingly hopeless struggle, and learn to enjoy REAL food again.

Before describing bodybuilding nutrition for losing excess fat weight while on your exercise program at "The Change Room" (you could call ANY good gym by this name!), it is necessary to first understand what you will be doing, and why you are doing it. In the final analysis, the physique you will have depends only on you, your knowledge, and your drive to achieve the ideal body you see in your mind. Do you have a visual image of how you want to look a year from now? No? – conjure one up, and work toward it.

Food is measured in calories. A calorie is the smallest unit of chemical energy that can be released as heat, or stored as fat, when food is metabolized by the body. It follows, then, that food which is high in calories is also high in energy value. Fats, for example, yield approximately 9 calories per gram, while protein and carbohydrates yield only 4 calories per gram. The energy we expend during work, exercise, and even at rest (it takes energy to breathe, grow hair and nails, pump blood, and keep warm enough) is also measured in calories—with vigorous activities using more calories than the more sedentary pastimes like reading, watching T.V., texting or Facebooking.

Only two things affect our bodyweight – the number of calories we take in as food and drink, and the number of calories we expend during work, exercise and rest. It is not necessary to count the calories in your food or compute how many you expend, from charts you could buy. Save your time and money. You need know only this:

If you take in more calories from your food than you expend during activity, the difference is stored as fat, on top of the muscles your body uses to move you around, and you look increasingly softer and rounder, or, "out of shape". The number your scale registers is going up. You suspect it is broken; in fact you are positive. Even your mirror is losing its fascination for you.

If you use up more calories during the day than you take in as food, especially if you are incorporating aerobics (much more on that later) into your health plan, your body begins to use the stored fat deposits for the energy it needs, and over time, as the fat gets used up, you lose size (and therefore, weight). The muscles, which were always there, begin to show and you look and feel healthier, more "in-shape". Narcissism may be your biggest problem soon, along with needing smaller clothing.

If you want visible muscle tone, you not only have to lose the fat that covers the muscles, but to strengthen and (usually) enlarge them as well, with progressive resistance weight training.

Before moving on to a more in-depth discussion of fats, protein and carbohydrates, there is another fact you should note. Some writers are now saying that certain individuals have a genetic predisposition to gaining excess weight in the form of fat. In other words, if your parents were obese, you have a better chance of being obese yourself, than if they weren't. Others believe that if a person's parents were obese, led sedentary lives, and knew virtually nothing about proper nutrition, then these lifestyle choices are likely to be embraced by their children. Is this "inherited" behaviour genetic or just bad luck in your choice of parents? I firmly side with the latter view, and have helped train many people away from their former unhealthy habits. Reduce your intake of food, increase your energy output with exercise and you will get smaller! Other reasons for staying fat are rationalizations and "cop-outs", and unfortunately there's no sugar-coated way to say it.

Weight is a mystery to some people. We've become slaves to the scale, that instrument that can weigh only mass—with no distinction between muscle and fat. The inadequacy of the scale becomes clear when we realize that muscle weighs at least twice as much as fat. For example, a piece of fat will weigh much less than a piece of red meat (muscle) that is the same size. When a person's body consists of lots of fat, say 35%, he or she can be the same height and weight as another whose body contains only 15% fat. The person with the higher fat content will be larger because fat displaces more volume (i.e. is less dense).

Therefore, it is not only possible, but probable, to reduce physical size, and gain weight, at the same time. This is because the muscles you are growing are denser than the fat you are shedding. If your goal is to reduce your size, forget your weight as measured on a scale, and get your positive reinforcement that changes are occurring by using a tape measure and a mirror. You will be cinching in your belt notch by notch. And you may weigh a little more!

I have had the pleasure of meeting, and being instructed by Lee Haney, a former Mr. Olympia (he won this most-coveted of bodybuilding awards several years in a row), and he recounts an interesting anecdote. At the time he was about 6'1" and weighed a rock-hard 250 pounds. He had cannonball shoulders and about a 28" waist – by his titles, he was acknowledged as the most physically impressive man on the planet. When he applied for a life insurance policy, it was denied, for according to actuarial tables, a 6'1" man who weighed 250 pounds HAD to be grossly overweight and thus a very poor risk from an insurance company's point of view. They couldn't see from his reported measurements that he had a body fat percentage of less than 5% and had a heart as strong as an ox. So weight as measured on a scale isn't always the best indicator of one's level of fitness or health. They lost a good policy.

The principles to remember at all times are:
1. Muscle weighs more than fat (it's denser).
2. A pound of muscle takes up less room on your body than a pound of fat.
3. Muscle is SHAPELY and fat is SHAPELESS.

What Does Your Body Need?

There is much talk about the need for a BALANCED diet. But what is it? Traditionally, most nutritionists define a balanced diet as eating from the five major food groups each day.

1. Meats, poultry (including eggs), fish
2. Milk and other dairy products (cheese, cottage cheese, yogurt).
3. Grains (breads and cereals).
4. Vegetables, fruits, legumes (peas, beans, lentils, soy beans), nuts
5. Fats (oils, butter, margarine).

This is a good system of eating for adequate health and for so-called "maintenance" diets—however, most of you who come to The Change Room want not so much to maintain your existing body weight and shape, as to change it. The body needs certain nutritional elements, but not necessarily at each meal.

People need protein (meat, eggs, milk, cheese, fish, poultry) for growth, maintenance, and tissue repair; vitamins and enzymes to act as catalysts in metabolic processes; and an energy source, which can be either fats (oils, butter, margarine) or carbohydrates (fruits, vegetables, grains, legumes, nuts and seeds). They also need minerals, water, and fiber. Each of these I will discuss briefly. Without energy, we do nothing, so—FATS FIRST.

Fats

This group includes butter, margarine, mayonnaise and other salad dressings, and all animal fats and vegetable oils. Serving sizes are not given for this group because these foods are not recommended for inclusion in a balanced diet. Some exceptions are vegetable oils, which provide some vitamin E and F; and butter and margarine which supply some vitamin A. You can **easily** get these elsewhere.

We get more than double the calories from the fat we eat, than we do from either protein or carbohydrates. Another way to put it is that a small amount of fatty food contains more calories than a large amount of "lean" food. Consider and remember the following values:

1 gram of fat   = 9 calories
1 gram of protein   = 4 calories
1 gram of carbohydrate   = 4 calories
1 gram of alcohol   = 8 calories (**nutrient-less**
                           carbohydrate)

While it is true that we need <u>some</u> fat in our diet (to carry the fat-soluble vitamins, and to make calcium available to the tissues, bones, and teeth), you would have to go to extremes to eat a <u>fat-deficient</u> diet, because fat is hidden in foods where you would never suspect it to be. For example, people think of pecans and peanuts as high-protein foods, whereas in fact, they contain a lot of fat and very little protein. A handful of peanuts is about 1/4 cup and contains 137 calories; of which 101 come from fat (~74% of the calories come from fat,—in pecans 90%). That's also why they taste so good, and therefore why it's so easy to overeat them. A medium-sized baked potato (5 oz or ~1/3 lb) has only 150 calories. Add a tablespoon of butter (100 calories/tbsp) and it jumps to 250 calories. Add another tablespoon of butter and a little sour cream (30 calories/tbsp) and you may have 380 calories. At that point, the potato itself is only 39% of the total calories,—yet many people blame the potato for being the fattening food.

Some people eliminate red meats (usually fairly high in fat – visibly marbled, or <u>not</u>), feeling that they can then eat more nuts. That just replaces one fat food with another. Others are proud that they have replaced butter, which is 100% fat, with margarine—which is also 100% fat. Except for the taste, you might as well pour on a little motor oil, or smear on some Vaseline; they're all 100% grease. By the way, have you ever noticed that if you leave margarine open on your counter, even flies won't land on it? They don't find it interesting as a nutrition source, but if you have a dog, you know that flies <u>will</u> land on anything HE manages to leave on your lawn. You do the math! So, **if you must**, choose a LITTLE butter.

As a population, we are so fat that it's a national disgrace. Fat people are prone to heart attack, diabetes, kidney disease, gallbladder problems, and a host of other medical problems. Fat people fill our hospitals. Obesity is our number one health problem, causing most of the others. The medical effects of a high-fat diet are devastating. Atherosclerosis and cancer of the colon have also been linked to high fat consumption. If these ailments do not concern you and all you really want is a slim figure, then decrease the fat in your diet anyway. You need no other reason than the awful number of calories that fat contains. It doesn't matter how you do it, but get the fat out. More on "HOW?" later, in Chapter 5.

For Those Wishing To Go A Little Deeper

Fats, like carbohydrates, consist of chains of carbon, hydrogen, and oxygen molecules. In food, fats contain relatively less oxygen than carbs. Therefore more oxidation is possible when the fat is consumed and metabolized within the body, with a greater potential for energy release. This is why fats contain more calories than either carbs or protein. As noted previously, one gram of fat releases 9 calories, while a gram of either protein or carbs will release only 4 calories.

Simple fats consist of one molecule of glycerol and up to 3 molecules of fatty acids. They make up 98% of the fat in food and in your body. Fatty acids are the components of fats which contain energy. Some fatty acid chains contain the maximum number of hydrogen atoms that the chain can hold, and are therefore called "saturated" fats. Others have missing hydrogen atoms, and are called "unsaturated' fats. Those missing many hydrogen atoms are called "polyunsaturated".

Fats that are liquid at room temperature are called oils and contain mostly unsaturated fatty acids. Oils are largely obtained from plant sources: safflower, corn, cottonseed, olive, soy bean, and peanut. Fats that are solid at room temperature are composed mostly of saturated fatty acids. These are usually of animal origin:

beef, pork, lamb, chicken, egg yolks, and cheese. Oil may be hardened by hydrogenation, whereby hydrogen is added to the fat molecule until the oil becomes solid at room temperature. Margarine is an example.

The body is able to synthesize fats from carbs or protein with the exception of linoleic acid. You need about 6 grams per day of this essential fatty acid, found mostly in vegetable oils.

Carbohydrates

Carbohydrates raise the blood-sugar level and supply the muscles with energy. They also help metabolize protein and fat. Bodybuilders say that fat burns in the flame of carbohydrates, so forget about any low-carb diet plans you may have heard about.
Without carbohydrates, fats could not be broken down in the liver, and digestive problems would occur. There are basically three kinds of carbohydrates.

1) Simple Carbohydrates
2) Processed Carbohydrates
3) Complex Carbohydrates

Simple Carbohydrates

These are single or double molecule sugars requiring little or no digestion. Hence, they enter the blood quickly, raising the concentration of blood sugar (glucose). Fructose, a simple sugar, occurs naturally in fruit and some vegetables, but in low concentrations. These foods are high in fiber, vitamins and minerals, and may be eaten **anytime** for a safe energy boost.

Processed Carbohydrates

These man-made "fruit substitutes" also provide you with a quick shot of immediate energy, and are found in candy, sugar, cake, ice cream, pastry, jams, jellies, syrups, sweet toppings, and other sweets. They have three major disadvantages, and therefore should be avoided like the plague. Unlike fruit, they contain no NUTRIENTS (vitamins), they often contain a lot of fat as well, and they contain none of fruit's fiber (cellulose) that is necessary for efficient elimination, intestinal cleansing and throughput. They provide only "empty" calories. Soft drinks are loaded with refined sugar and have no nutritional content at all. Acids such as citric acid or orthophosphoric acid are added to soft drinks to keep the sugar in solution. These substances destroy tooth enamel and injure the stomach lining. Your dentist owes a large part of his income to processed carbohydrates. Avoid them.

When your body detects the huge and sudden rise in your blood sugar level caused by eating these "sweets", the pancreas secretes insulin into the bloodstream to counteract it, and your blood sugar level drops dramatically. That high-energy feeling is replaced by a feeling of weakness and fatigue. To stay "up", you are drawn to another "fix" of processed sugar (I'll just have one more "brownie"—thanks!). The result is overeating of processed sugars—which are very high in calories—and weight gain. Again, avoid these substances as you would fat, if you want that slimmer, lithe physique. This leaves us with one main source for our energy requirements, the often-shunned complex carbohydrates.

Complex Carbohydrates

Vegetables and whole grains contain "complex" long-chained carbohydrate molecules. Such carbohydrates provide gradually released energy, because they require prolonged enzymatic action to be broken down into the simple sugars for digestion. Their chief value over the simple carbohydrates of fruit is their ability to provide a continual energy supply due to this gradual release. Since digestion may take hours, glucose is released slowly into the blood. Consequently, insulin is also released slowly to properly regulate your blood sugar level. This keeps your energy high for a longer period of time, and suppresses hunger, which is triggered by low blood sugar. For this reason, fruit before a workout would be good, but the energy might not last for 1-1½ hours, whereas the energy derived from beans or pasta probably will sustain a solid, lengthy workout. Both together would be best.

The most <u>concentrated</u> form of complex carbohydrate is starch. It comprises about 70% of wheat, rice, corn, millet, buckwheat, spelt, quinoa, pasta, cous cous, oatmeal . . . . . (grains), and about 40% of peas and various beans (legumes).

Both simple and complex carbohydrates are converted into glucose, which is used by the brain, the nervous system and the muscles. Some of it is stored, for reserve energy, in the muscles and liver as glycogen. <u>Excess</u> glucose is turned into fatty acids and stored as bodyfat. Since the glycogen deposits are usually full, most of the excess simple sugars are stored as fat. This is why simple sugars are so devastating to a dieter. Sugar puts your body in a fat storage mode, storing not just the calories from the sugar itself, but a good deal of the calories from the rest of the meal as well! Hence, it is important not to eat excess carbohydrates when the goal is weight (fat) loss. When caloric intake is reduced, the body reconverts the fat into glucose to be used as fuel for energy. It is "burned up," and excess body fat is reduced – along with weight. This process occurs most readily when weight training (anaerobic activity) is combined with cardiovascular activity (aerobic activity), usually on alternate days. I like to train in this manner, taking 1 day per week "off" to do other types of activity.

Complex carbohydrates contribute to physical stamina and mental stability, and are the body's most efficient and low-calorie source of energy. They have another huge plus going for them – they contain FIBER.

Fiber

Fiber (or roughage) is the indigestible part of plant tissue made up of cellulose, lignin, and pectin. It is a type of complex carbohydrate requiring a special enzyme for digestion which humans cannot make. For this reason, it contains no usable calories and does not break down in the body – it just moves through as indigestible "bulk", scrubbing its way along to the exit and taking some fat along with it. It gives the intestinal wall something substantial to push through the system as it contracts.

Fiber thus aids elimination by increasing the rate of food transit through the digestive system and prevents constipation.

Insufficient dietary fiber has been implicated in such diseases as diverticulitis, colonic cancer, diabetes, cardiovascular disease, hemorrhoids and varicose veins. Adequate fiber is absolutely essential for intestinal and overall health. Cholesterol deposits in the bloodstream are responsible for causing heart attacks, and it has been shown that serum cholesterol can be significantly reduced by increasing the fiber content of foods back to what it was before refined carbs (carbohydrates) became so popular. High fiber foods take up a lot of room in the stomach, but yield few calories for their bulk. An apple contains less than 100 calories, whereas a piece of pecan pie explodes with 688 calories.

Fiber creates a functional decrease of fat intake in two ways: it speeds removal of waste so less fat can be absorbed, and it binds with fat molecules, rendering them insoluble, therefore unavailable for absorption.

Most fruits and vegetables are high in fiber, as are nuts, seeds, legumes, and whole grains. Raw wheat bran may be sprinkled over cereal or other foods. Have a large raw salad daily as insurance against fiber and mineral deficiency. Include a wide variety of raw vegetables in your salad, not just lettuce and tomato. Try to make it colorful.

Protein

Proteins are the fundamental structural components of all living cells. Less the weight of your bones and water, about 86% of the body is protein. Enzymes and many hormones are protein. In order to build up, maintain and repair body tissue, we require protein, water and minerals. In the event of insufficient protein intake, the body will not grow, and established tissues will atrophy.

Muscle tissue is composed of 75% water and 25% protein, yet it is the protein that allows the muscle to hold fluid, and gives it the ability to contract. The skin and nails are protein. They form a waterproof, protective covering for the body. Protein, forming the walls of blood vessels, renders them elastic. The oxygen-carrying hemoglobin in blood is protein, and so are the antibodies that fight bacterial and viral infections. Bones and teeth are mostly mineral, but it is a protein based matrix that forms their foundation.

Protein molecules consists of smaller components, or building blocks called amino acids, which are long chains of carbon, hydrogen, oxygen, and nitrogen molecules, sometimes with certain minerals added. Protein foods are broken down by digestion into their constituent amino acids. They then enter the bloodstream, are distributed throughout the body and reassembled into the different protein based tissues. Isn't that incredible? In order for the body to make protein, 22 different amino acids must be present simultaneously, and in the correct proportions to one another by weight. Of these 22 amino acids, 14 can be manufactured by the body from carbs, and are called *nonessential*. The remaining 8 cannot be made in the body, and are termed *essential* amino acids. If any one of the 8 essential amino acids is missing, no protein can be synthesized. The remaining amino acids are then converted to fat or carbs and either stored or used for energy.

A protein food that contains all of the essential amino acids in correct proportion to one another is a complete, or balanced protein. Animal based proteins are balanced. Foods from plant sources such as vegetables, grains and fruit are deficient in one or more of the essential amino acids and are not balanced.

Foods of plant origin MAY be balanced by eating them in combinations that complement one another. For example, you may combine corn, which is low in tryptophan and high in methionine (essential amino acids), with beans, which are low in methionine and high in tryptophan. The combination yields balanced protein nearly as high in quality as steak, but it is low in fat and calories, and has complex carbs and fiber. It's not necessary to know the names of all the amino acids, but you should know how to combine plant proteins to balance them. Nor is it necessary to become a vegetarian. You can still eat meat to add variety to your meals.

The following 4 groupings of foods will help you to choose foods that will complement one another in this way. Choose between adjacent categories only. For example, grains and legumes will provide complete protein, but grains and seeds will not. Milk products and eggs are complete by themselves, but have an abundance of certain amino acids that will improve the balance of grains.

  A) DAIRY PRODUCTS—eggs, milk, cottage cheese, cheese, yogurt
  B) GRAINS—wheat, rye, rice, corn, oats, millet, barley, buckwheat, quinoa, bulgar wheat, cous cous, breads, cereals, and pasta
  C) LEGUMES – soy beans, navy beans, lima beans, kidney beans, pea beans, broad beans, black beans, lentils, chick peas, peas, black eye peas, split peas, peanuts
  D) SEEDS – sesame, sunflower, pumpkin, squash

Nitrogen Balance

Nitrogen, a major component of protein, enters your system in the food you eat, and leaves as the end product of protein metabolism. When nitrogen input exceeds output, the body is said to be in "positive nitrogen balance". This means that protein based tissues are being formed (which absolutely includes muscle tissue), and that the body is growing. This occurs during childhood, pregnancy, and recovery from illness or injury, but only with adequate protein intake. An athlete deliberately developing bigger muscles must also be in a state of positive nitrogen balance.

Negative nitrogen balance occurs when nitrogen output exceeds input. Protein based body tissues are being broken down faster than they are being replaced. This happens when protein intake is low, or is of poor quality (amino acid imbalance). It also occurs during illness or injury, acute pain, and interrupted sleep patterns. Such emotional stresses such as anger, fear, or anxiety stimulate the secretion of adrenaline, resulting in nitrogen loss. It is impossible to build or even maintain protein based tissue (muscle tissue) during negative nitrogen balance.

For bodybuilding purposes, eggs are the number-one protein; milk proteins are number-two; fish, meat and poultry proteins are number-three.

Protein in the body is in a constant state of exchange (into energy, for tissue maintenance and growth, and for recuperation from activity) and must be replaced regularly if muscular gains are to be realized. To flood the tissues with a constant supply of protein, it would be necessary to eat protein foods in small quantities on an almost continuous basis. Since this is impractical for most people (and high in calories), most serious trainers try to consume about 5 or 6 nutrient and "protein-dense" small meals per day, some of them merely amino-acid (protein powder) supplements. More on supplements in Chapter 3.

Some experts say that an adult can subsist well on a minimum of ½—1 gram of protein per kilogram of bodyweight, and this may be true of sedentary individuals. However, athletes in heavy training to increase muscular mass need at least 2-3 grams (or more) of protein per kilogram of bodyweight. For example, a 220 lb. man (100 kg) would need around 200 grams of protein per day while training hard.

Since the body can only use about 25-30 grams of protein every 3 hours (without excreting any excess), he would need about 6 or 7 small meals throughout the day, each containing about 30 grams of protein, and enough complex carbohydrates to sustain his energy without gaining (fat) weight. Gaining muscular weight is not only OK, but is in fact, the goal, as fat stores decrease. Your protein meals should be small, and frequent.

Here's where that protein could come from:

Food Source	Quantity	Protein (g)	Approximate Quantity to Yield 30 grams
Fish	1 lb.	120	4 oz.
Cheese	1 lb.	112	4 oz.
Lean beef	1 lb.	100	5 oz.
Turkey	1 lb.	92	5 oz.
Chicken	1 lb.	80	6 oz.
Heart	1 lb.	77	6 oz.

Tuna (canned)	1 can	30	1 can
Cottage cheese	1 cup	30	1 cup
Milk	1 cup	9	3 cups
Egg	1	7	4

Even if your protein intake is sufficient, your body can still be in negative nitrogen balance if your caloric intake is too low. The body will chemically strip the nitrogen bearing amino acid group away from the protein molecule, and excrete it in the form of urea. The remaining carbon chain may then be burned for energy. What is happening is that protein in your meals is being used for energy instead of carbs and fat. If the protein intake is also low, then protein based tissues (muscle tissue) will be broken down to provide energy. Energy needs take precedence over tissue maintenance.

Ketosis

Carbs and fats are said to be protein sparing foods. They prevent the use of protein for energy. Fats alone will not spare protein, because fatty acids cannot be converted into glucose. The brain runs on glucose and oxygen, and must have them continuously. It uses up to 2/3 of all blood glucose, mostly from carbs. Amino acids can be changed into glucose, but less effectively. This is why a low carb diet causes fatigue, weakness, and dizziness. Therefore, even on a weight reduction diet, sufficient carbs must be supplied to spare protein and maintain a proper blood sugar level.

When carb intake is very low, the body will use either stored fat or dietary fat for energy, depending on caloric intake. Some of the fatty acids are not completely burned, however, and form keto acids in your blood, a condition known as ketosis. In this state, large amounts of nitrogen and salts are lost in the urine. Ketosis makes the blood acidic, which contributes to the symptoms of fatigue, irritability, and insomnia. Not good at all! You can test for ketosis by using Ketostix, which are available at most drugstores.

When there are ketone bodies in your system, the test sticks will turn purple when they come in contact with your urine.

To help guide you in determining the minimum amount of carbohydrate you should have in your diet, gradually cut down on carbs and test occasionally for ketosis. When you finally see the sticks start to turn purple, increase the amount of carbs until the ketone reaction ceases. This level of monitoring for carbs is usually for pre-contest bodybuilders only. For the rest of us, just don't go on extremely low-carb diets, EVER.

The diet should provide a minimum allowance of protein for growth and maintenance of tissues, plus some extra amount for insurance. Hard work does NOT require extra protein, just extra energy, because the body becomes accustomed to the work load, and does not need to grow. However, an athlete in heavy training does require more protein because he is constantly increasing (incrementally) the work load in order to stimulate the growth of new muscle tissue. He wants to get bigger.

Cholesterol

Many people worry about eating eggs because of the cholesterol they contain (the average egg contains about 250 mg). Studies have yet to find a single bodybuilder in normal good health, who eats large quantities of raw eggs, and has an elevated cholesterol count because of it. Doctors interested in the prevention and treatment of cardiovascular disease have long ago discarded the theory that animal fat is the cause of heart disease. A little-recognized fact is that the body itself manufactures more cholesterol daily, than you could ever possibly eat. The body reduces cholesterol output or produces more, depending on how much of it you ingest. Dr. John Yudkin, Professor Emeritus of Nutrition at the University of London, explains that there is no sure link established between diet and coronary thrombosis. The triglyceride level in the blood is a much better indicator of coronary risk than cholesterol. The blood triglyceride, he says, is determined by how much sugar, not how many eggs (the cholesterol in the yolks) you eat. This is yet another good reason to stay away from processed carbohydrates.

Since eggs have been mentioned, let's take it one step further. If a trainer wants to eat four eggs to get a 28 gram protein hit, he would be well-advised to blend them RAW (uncooked) in some low-fat milk with some fresh fruit. The lecithin that occurs naturally in the yolk of the egg serves to emulsify the cholesterol, and no cooking preserves the protein intact. Cooking of eggs renders the lecithin useless, you still get the cholesterol, and some of the protein is denatured (rendered inassimilable) in the process. The protein in an egg is divided between the yolk and the white, but all the minerals and vitamins are in the yolk, along with the fat. Eggs are rich in phosphorus, sulfur, iron and Vitamin A. If you can't stand the thought of consuming raw eggs (especially "invisible" in a blended shake), then poach them very lightly to get the most good from them.

Vitamins And Minerals

It was noted earlier in this chapter that our bodies need vitamins and minerals in addition to protein, and carbohydrates. It is important for bodybuilders to have some basic knowledge of the main vitamins and minerals, and this follows. Those who want more specific knowledge on individual vitamins and minerals should study books on nutrition or see a nutritionist. I will include a chart at the end of this chapter that will tell you some of the best foods from which to get your vitamins and minerals.

Vitamins are organic compounds, meaning that they are based on carbon, and originate from living tissue. Plants can make the vitamins we need; humans cannot. Vitamins act as catalysts: they promote a chemical reaction without taking part in it, and without being used up. This is why vitamins are needed in such small amounts. Vitamins themselves do not yield energy, but help to extract energy from fats and carbs. They help to synthesize bone and tissue without becoming part of these structures. Vitamins fall into two categories: fat soluble and water soluble.

Vitamins A, D, E, and K are fat soluble, meaning that they will dissolve in fat but not in water. Consequently, they are found in fatty foods such as cream, butter, meats, fish fat (oils) and vegetable fat (oils). Since they are insoluble in water, these vitamins cannot be passed in the urine. They are stored, mainly in the liver, and may accumulate to toxic levels if too many A or D supplements are taken. Since they are stored for long periods, a deficiency may take time to reveal itself. Linoleic acid, an essential fatty acid, is sometimes called vitamin F.

Vitamins B and C are water soluble. They are NOT stored in the body, and are excreted in the urine and perspiration. For these reasons, any deficiency will quickly show up. Since they pass rapidly through the body, these vitamins do not accumulate in toxic amounts. Bioflavenoids, which assist vitamin C, are often called vitamin P.

Minerals are found in every cell in the body, not only as catalysts, but also as components of hard and soft tissue, and body fluids. The body cannot synthesize minerals; they must be supplied by the diet.

Vitamins

Vitamin A	is important for good vision, promotes growth and maintenance of tissues, bone, teeth, skin, hair, mucous membranes, fights infection, aids digestion.
Vitamin B Complex	(12 B vitamins) is involved in just about every bodily function, and is especially essential in cell growth, red blood cell production, and the metabolism of fats, sugars, carbohydrates and protein; maintenance of the nervous system, eyes, hair, skin, mouth, liver, digestive system; fighting stress. All the B complex vitamins must be taken at once because they work together. Sugar, alcohol and coffee deplete the B complex vitamins. They are lost in urine and perspiration.

Vitamin C Complex (including the bioflavenoids or Vitamin P) is a great detoxifier, stress fighter and healing agent. An antioxidant, vitamin C protects vitamins A, B complex and E against oxidation. It helps form collagen, a protein found in skin, ligaments, tendons and bone; helps build red blood cells; fights allergy and infection, including colds. It is essential for the proper absorption of minerals, especially calcium. It helps promote workout recovery, prevents capillary damage and sore muscles.

Vitamin D helps the body to utilize calcium and phosphorus. Both are required for growth of bones and teeth, and for heart, blood and nerve activity. Sunlight will synthesize vitamin D in the oil of the skin. It works together with vitamin A.

Vitamin E is another antioxidant that protects vitamins A, B, and C.
It allows the blood to carry more oxygen; helps prevent blood clots; improves muscular and heart endurance; helps prevent heart disease. Although fat soluble, excess vitamin E is passed in the urine, and leaves the body within 3 days.

Vitamin F 3 of the fatty acids (linoleic, linolenic, arachidonic) are essential for cell structure; glandular activity; blood coagulation; healthy skin, hair and nerves; help control cholesterol deposits in arteries, and help the body utilize calcium, phosphorus, and vitamin A.

<u>Vitamin K</u>	is important in blood clotting, carbohydrate metabolism and liver function. Cultured milk products aid the intestinal bacteria in producing this vitamin.
<u>Vitamin P</u>	bioflavenoids are found in the same sources as vitamin C and work with it to strengthen blood vessels, maintain collagen, and fight infection. Vitamin C and P deficiency may increase the tendency to bleed or bruise easily.

Minerals

Your body also needs adequate amounts of the following minerals for good health: calcium, magnesium, phosphorus, iron, iodine, potassium, zinc, manganese, and sodium, as well as small amounts of trace minerals like selenium, cobalt, and chromium. They occur in small quantities in your food, but if you buy supplements as insurance against mineral deficiencies in your diet, make sure they are "chelated." Otherwise, your body will not absorb them properly. Chelation (pronounced "key-lation") increases absorption of the minerals by 20-25%.

As a group of compounds, minerals (including metallic and non-metallic trace elements) are vital because:

1. They maintain both electrical and acid/base balances.
2. They maintain proper cellular pressure.
3. They assist in conducting nerve impulses.
4. They stimulate or inhibit enzyme actions.
5. They are actual structural elements in the body, in bones, teeth, tendons, and cartilage.

Although each mineral has many different functions, I'll just touch briefly on those functions which directly affect your training.

<u>Iron</u>	is found in the blood's hemoglobin. It is involved in the carrying of elemental oxygen in red blood cells. No oxygen = no training. It is used in protein metabolism, respiration and growth.
	Note: If you supplement with iron, take it separately from Vitamin E or any fish oils you may be taking. The effects of these substances tend to cancel one another.
<u>Calcium</u>	The body contains more calcium than any other mineral, mostly in the bones and teeth. Calcium promotes muscle growth and contraction and is vital for the functioning of nerve cells and enzyme activity. It is also responsible for transmission of impulses from nerves to muscles.
<u>Phosphorus</u>	works along with calcium, and is found in every cell in the body. It is used for protein, carbohydrate and fat metabolism; is a main component of strong bones, and at the cellular level it is a major component of ATP, the form of energy used by muscles. Protein foods are high in phosphorus.
<u>Zinc</u>	is needed for growth, insulin and protein synthesis; is required to help certain enzymes prevent the build-up of lactic acid (the substance in your cells that causes that burning sensation near the end of a set of repetitions) in muscles.

Magnesium	all enzymes needed for the metabolism of ATP (adenosine triphosphate) for muscular energy require magnesium. It also regulates body heat, contraction of muscles and the synthesis of body proteins. Don't go without this one! Deficiency symptoms include tremors, quivering, and muscular cramping.
Selenium	helps detoxify contaminants in the environment, and helps protect you against cancer and other diseases.
Iodine	is an essential component of the thyroid gland, which controls protein synthesis, carbohydrate absorption, metabolism and intellect. All seafood is rich in iodine.
Potassium	is found in the fluid within the cells. Muscles, including the heart, cannot contract without this electrolyte to carry nerve signals. Deficiencies are particularly serious to people "working out". Irregular heartbeat, cessation of muscular contractions, and the abnormal conduction of nerve impulses can devastate your training program. Since active people have greater needs for potassium (because potassium is lost in sweat), they should be aware that continued (or frequent) muscle cramping can be an early sign of a deficiency.
Cobalt	Vitamin B_{12} needs cobalt to carry out its biochemical functions. If you supplement with iron, you may also need more cobalt to maintain a proper ratio of both.

Silicon	This mineral is related to the mineralization and calcification of bone tissue. Your sand-eating child is trying to get some!
Manganese	Enzymes containing manganese are very active in the mitochondria, the "powerhouses" of the cell, where energy production occurs. It is also a vital component of enzymes involved in carbohydrate and fat metabolism.
Chromium	is an essential mineral for humans. It is used to make Glucose Tolerance Factor (GTF), which is important to insulin function. Insulin helps in fat metabolism (breakdown) and protein synthesis (growth). Food processing and refining reduces the amounts found in "natural" food. GO NATURAL wherever possible!!
Sodium	another important electrolyte necessary for nerve and muscle function, sodium is the most common mineral nutrient in your diet. It assists digestion and is the main source of fluid regulation within the body. Other functions include the maintenance of blood chemistry balance, and purification of the body from poisonous carbon dioxide.

Sodium

Lack of sodium is not a problem in the modern world. There is sodium (we normally only think of it in the form of sodium chloride, or table salt) in virtually every food in its natural state. Tap water contains sodium! Most people ingest 3-7 grams of sodium a day, 3-5 times the ideal amount. Its "downside'" is that it causes the body to retain water, up to 30 times its weight, causing bloating and driving up blood pressure. Some of what people call their fat is a certain amount of fluid retention, caused by the chronic use of too much salt. Cut way back, and some of your so-called "fat" will be secreted almost immediately. The scale will register a weight loss, but it won't necessarily be all from fat – but so??? Even excess water takes up space, on your frame, and in your clothes.

Muscular, lean bodies don't need <u>excess</u> sodium. **Never** use table salt. Hide the shaker. Stay away from salty snacks (I was going to say "as much as possible" but you might take that as a loophole!). You will soon get to like the taste of unsalted food. The list of high-sodium foods is endless, but here are some of the main offenders. Remember, you can "safely" have about 2 g (2000 mg) per <u>day</u>. **PER DAY!!!**

Amount	Food	Milligrams of Sodium
1 tsp	Table salt	2000 (i.e. 2g)
1 cup	Chow Mein	1675
1 cup	Cottage cheese	900
1	Pickle	930
1 cup	Soup, canned (avg.)	1000
1 cup	Tomato juice	875

By means of contrast, here are some low-sodium foods.

Amount	Food	Milligrams of Sodium
1 ear	Cob of corn	1
1	Baked potato	5
4 oz.	Skinned white chicken	87
1	Large apple	2
½	Cantaloupe	24
1	Large pear	1
1	Large orange	0

Limit your sodium intake to foods that naturally contain sodium; avoid canned food <u>completely</u> (sodium is used here in large quantities, as a preservative). Read labels, and if a lot of salt is listed, at least drain and rinse the product before consuming it.

Fresh foods are always best, but if time and convenience demand the intake of prepared foods, use frozen rather than canned. There are 450 mg of sodium in a cup of <u>canned</u> peas and carrots, but only 50 mg in a cup of <u>frozen</u> peas and carrots.

While I'm on the subject of avoiding all forms of preservatives, which are fairly toxic to the body in the quantities food manufacturers use, here's a shopping tip. Most grocery stores have their meat section along one side, the dairy section along the back and the produce department along the other side. All the aisles contain canned foods, and foods wrapped in waxed paper, cardboard, foil wrap and/or cellophane. To keep these "aisle" foods saleable indefinitely, they are <u>loaded</u> with salt and various other unpronounceable preservatives and chemicals (as a rule of thumb, if you can't pronounce some of the ingredients on a label, don't buy that product). Shop down one side, across the back of the store, back the other side, and pay at the front. Avoid the aisles <u>completely</u>.

Except for cat food. Unless, of course, you want your cat to be healthy, too.

<u>Water</u>

As 45% to 60% of the body is water, it is obviously essential to life. It regulates body temperature and is involved in the vast majority of the body's metabolic processes. Most importantly for trainers striving to reduce their body fat percentage, water aids fat mobilization and utilization, aids in recuperation, flushes the system of toxins, and increases filtration by the kidneys.

Since water is lost rapidly during both aerobic activity (especially) and weight training (whether or not you visibly sweat), it is necessary to consume plenty each day. The rate of turnover is about 6% of total body water per day. A minimum of 5-6 glasses is recommended daily. Some of this may be milk, tea, coffee, or soup, but most of it should be pure water. Carry a water bottle with you everywhere, and "stay hydrated". It will even decrease hunger somewhat, so don't forget your regular feedings.

Hard water (usually comes from deep wells through limestone) is fine to drink. If your water is "hard", it has dissolved minerals in it (mainly calcium). It's the calcium that sometimes appears as white spots on glassware left to dry in the dish rack. Softened water is high in sodium, because water softeners work by exchanging sodium for the calcium. Try to avoid drinking softened water; remember the section on sodium?

Remember that most foods are largely composed of water, so hunger is often confused with thirst. We think we are hungry, when the body is actually craving water. Give yourself a low-calorie break and drink plenty <u>between meals</u>. Excess fluid intake at meals should be avoided, since it dilutes the digestive juices. Apples and other juicy fruits contain lots of water. The next time you feel hungry between meals, ask yourself if you are hungry enough to eat an apple. If the answer is yes, go ahead and eat one. If the answer is no, you aren't hungry, you are bored. Go for a walk, and take your water bottle along with you!

Sources of Vitamins and Minerals

We mentioned previously that vitamins come in two varieties, water soluble (vitamins B, C, and P), and fat soluble (vitamins A, D, E and K). If you buy them in supplement form, the water soluble ones will be tablets, and the fat soluble ones will be in liquid form within gelatin capsules.

Water Soluble Vitamins

<u>B-Complex</u>		brewer's yeast, liver, whole grain cereals eggs, poultry, green vegetables, fish, fruit
B_1	Thiamine	wheat germ, bran, blackstrap molasses
B_2	Riboflavin	organ meats—tongue, kidneys, liver, heart
B_3	Niacinamide	wheat germ, peanuts, lean meat

	Choline	wheat germ, lecithin, egg yolks
B_5	Pantothenic acid	organ meats, yolks, whole grain cereals
B_6	Pyridoxine	wheat germ, bananas, meats
B_7	Biotin	soy beans, egg yolks, brown rice
B_8	Inosital	citrus fruits, (unprocessed) raw grains
B_9	Folic acid	leafy green vegetables
B_{10}	PABA	wheat germ, liver, yeast, molasses
B_{12}	Cobalamin	fish, dairy products
B_{13}	Orotic acid	brewer's yeast
B_{15}	Pangamic acid	liver, whole grain products

Vitamin C	- ascorbic acid	citrus fruits, pineapple, cantaloupe, turnips, cabbage, spinach, green peppers, tomatoes, green vegetables, most fresh fruits and vegetables
Vitamin F		soy bean, wheat germ, corn, sunflower, safflower and cod liver oils
Vitamin P	- bioflavenoids	buckwheat, lemons, grapefruit
	- (for use with C)	grapes, plums, cherries

Fat Soluble Vitamins

Vitamin A	yellow fruits, yellow vegetables, tomatoes, spinach, dairy products, eggs, liver, fish, carrots, fish liver oils
Vitamin D	fish liver oils, fish, sunlight, yolks, milk
Vitamin E	wheat germ or its oil, molasses, raw nuts, leafy vegetables, legumes, seeds
Vitamin K	citrus fruits, green peppers, liver, egg yolks, molasses, vegetable oils

Minerals

Calcium	dairy, shellfish, green vegetables, grains
Chromium	liver, whole grains, yeast, vegetable oil, meats
Copper	liver, whole grains, seafood, green vegetables
Iron	liver, eggs, lean meat, whole bread, vegetables
Magnesium	nuts, legumes, soy, dark green vegetables, apple
Manganese	wheat germ, sunflower seeds, legumes
Phosphorus	seeds, grains, nuts, poultry, fish, meats
Selenium	broccoli, tuna, onions, bran, tomatoes
Potassium	bananas, grains, potato peels, oranges
Zinc	beans, seeds, nuts, liver, yeast, wheat germ
Iodine	all seafood, fish liver oil, kelp, iodized salt
Sodium	everywhere, even tap water, table salt

SO folks, you probably are seeing a pattern above, namely that a few of the most common foods provide many of your daily required vitamins and minerals.

To get all of them from the above listings, you need to incorporate the following foods into your daily eating program.

Vegetables - yellow, green, leafy, red . . . .
Citrus fruits
Whole grains, nuts and seeds
Wheat germ, fish liver oil, organ meats (liver, heart, kidneys, gizzards)

Uncooked eggs (especially the yolks)
Lean meat - beef, chicken, fish

The following natural "supplements" make great additions to your program.

<u>Alfalfa sprouts</u> supply Vitamin K, calcium, and almost all the vitamins and minerals.
<u>Molasses</u> supplies calcium, iron, potassium, B vitamins, vitamin E, copper, magnesium and phosphorus.
<u>Lecithin</u> supplies phosphorus, and helps with digestion of fat.
<u>Brewer's yeast</u> supplies the B vitamins, many minerals and amino acids.

I'll go into supplements a little more in-depth in Chapter 3.

CHAPTER 3 Supplements -
Are They Necessary?

Many individuals come into the gym overweight, saying that they want to "tone-up," or point to a 20 pound protruding belly, saying "I just want to get rid of this." If this, or a variation of these statements, sounds familiar to you, you must understand the following:

BODYBUILDING, TONING UP, SIZE REDUCTION ETC . . .

IS AT LEAST 50% NUTRITION.

These individuals assume exercise is the "cure-all" for all problems, and proceed to train without paying any attention to their diet. This is a common occurrence, especially among beginners.

It is quite possible to work out diligently for a year (or two!) without good results. You can have rock-hard obliques (the muscles on the sides of your waist) and "washboard" abs but they will never be noticed if they're covered by a thick (or even a thin) fat layer! In order to succeed, you will have to be just as dedicated to your diet as you are to your training.

The reason for taking food supplements is that most people (including bodybuilders) have been on poor diets for so long that their systems are imbalanced. The food you eat may not contain enough nutrients (vitamins, minerals, proteins etc.) to keep the body's endocrine system (it produces growth and other hormones) in balance, thus keeping you from the growth you expect after each workout. You can upgrade the quality of the food you eat and still be short of the proper nutrients in the proper amounts, because training increases your body's needs for them. You could get more nutrients by eating a lot more good food, but the extra calories would be hard to work off. Hence, these nutrients must be supplied by food supplements.

However, it's not simply a matter of gulping down a few supplements with your meals for you to be instantly in proper balance. It takes time, usually 4-6 weeks. For best long-term results, supplements should be taken for 3 days and then stopped for 3 days, which allows maximum utilization of the supplement without toxifying the system.

Anyone who wants to maximize their gains (fat loss and muscle gain) must first get on a good all-round nutritional program, with all the necessary elements to feed the system. Once in balance, advanced supplements are necessary to get the system operating at peak efficiency. When this state is achieved, you should see gains from nearly every workout—more repetitions, more weight used, body fat levels decreasing, lean body mass increasing, better posture and flexibility, higher all-round energy, and the increased self-esteem that these physical changes bring. How badly do you want this? Really?? Then read on.

The role, and sources, of vitamins has already been discussed, and you should probably take a one-a-day vitamin/mineral tablet, even when you are eating optimally. There are other supplements, both natural and man-made that you can take, and a discussion of the most popular ones follows.

The bodybuilder's goal of increased muscular size and body fat reduction can only be achieved when the body's glands are healthy and hormone production is in a state of "positive nitrogen balance". Bodybuilders have taken anabolic steroids and synthetic testosterone (synthetic male sex hormones) for years as a means of increasing protein synthesis (muscle gains), but the effects of steroids are only temporary, and potentially disastrous or fatal. It is a common assumption that those who take steroids "magically" turn into muscular hulks, despite the known risks. Nothing could be further from the truth. If that were so, 99.9% of serious gym ironheads would look like the current Mr. Olympia. You know they don't. Steroids certainly enhance a person's ability to recuperate between workouts, but those workouts are brutal and frequent, often twice per day, and would be enough to almost kill a normal individual (that would be you and me!).

The glands within your body are capable of manufacturing hormones naturally, but ONLY if all the right nutrients are available to nourish them. When glandular imbalances occur, as evidenced by hard workouts but no gains, corrective measures must be taken. You will need to follow a high-protein diet of hormone-precursing foods and supplements (those that provide the building blocks the body uses to produce the required hormones). In other words, if you want to build a wall, you need to provide not only enough, but the right kind of building blocks. It's the same with muscle cells.

Natural Supplements

Some of the natural hormone precursors include: wheat germ oil, kelp, alfalfa, Brewer's yeast, vitamin B complex, vitamin C complex, vitamin E, the herb ginseng, and raw eggs.

Wheat Germ Oil — is very rich in vitamins A, B, and E, iron, and the necessary unsaturated fatty acids. It has anti-stress and endurance factors that enable people to better handle hard training. It is best taken on an empty stomach immediately after a work out.

Kelp — is a salt water plant which contains 44 minerals and is especially high in iodine, a major part of the thyroid hormone. Too much can depress thyroid function, which is fat and carbohydrate metabolism. It tastes horrible to me, but you can gulp it down quickly. You won't take too much!

Alfalfa — is 20% protein and contains all 8 essential amino acids, plus 8 enzymes necessary for food digestion. It also contains many minerals and trace elements, and is the richest source of calcium known, especially important during high-protein diets. You can buy alfalfa and sprout it yourself, then put it in salads, or buy it already sprouted in the fresh vegetable section of your store.

<u>Brewer's Yeast</u>	contains almost no fat, starch, or sugar, but has excellent protein (37% compared to 23% in meat), 17 different vitamins including the complete B complex, 16 amino acids, iron, selenium and several other important minerals. It helps to slow the aging process (sure it does!) and to recharge worn-out cells. It tastes pretty bad, so hide a couple of teaspoonfuls in a heavily flavored protein shake.
<u>Ginseng</u>	The Siberian variety has been used by the Chinese for centuries. Its fans claim that it helps the body cope with stress, normalizes hormone levels, reduces fatigue, reduces cholesterol, treats insomnia, depression, diabetes, impotence . . . . I took 2 tablets each day last week, and now I have 14 less tablets.

Lipotropic Supplements

When dieting to lose fat, the use of lipotropic or fat burning agents is helpful. They don't perform miracles, but they do speed up results, especially when coupled with a diet that is low in fat. The main lipotropics are the B vitamins choline and inositol (B_8), which aid in the production of lecithin. These substances enable the liver and gall bladder to metabolize fats more readily and efficiently. 250-1000 mg is recommended with meals (if you can afford it).

Other lipotropics that could be taken are the amino acid methionine, vitamin C complex, B complex, kelp, alfalfa, brewer's yeast tablets, and fish oils (halibut liver oil and cod liver oil). These oils, rich in vitamins A and D, help to reduce arthritis pain and inflammation, possibly helping to relieve the pain, inflammation and mild tendonitis that often accompanies moderate to heavy weight training.

Protein Supplements

One of the wonderful benefits considered to be a "spin-off" of the 1960s race to put a man on the moon was the development of powdered food. The astronauts couldn't take, prepare or do the clean-up of meals comprised of steak and vegetables etc., so intensive research began to find out just how much of "normal" food was <u>actually essential</u> to keep people alive and alert for many days at a time so far away from home. Not only were the biochemists involved in this research successful, they were successful "in spades". The astronauts performed their tasks admirably and came back healthy. Companies soon realized that this method of eating could be used by the entire planet-bound population, and powdered supplements (now called meal replacements) began to be promoted and marketed, especially by weight loss companies. Stripping away everything but the protein component of such products has led to the protein powder industry, and they are now used extensively by all serious bodybuilders as an addition to their diets, with or between the normal meals. Most of them are comprised of protein from milk and eggs, and/or soy isolates, as sources.

It was stated earlier that the body must be in a constant state of "positive nitrogen balance" in order to enhance muscular gains. You are already getting lots of protein from the traditional sources: beef, pork, fish, eggs, chicken, milk and soy beans. Soy beans?? Read on.

Vegetarian bodybuilders know all about soy protein. So do bodybuilders who suffer from lactose intolerance, the impaired ability to digest milk and milk-based products.

Soy beans, soy milk and tofu digests almost exactly the same way beef protein does. Other studies done comparing soy protein with eggs and milk yield similar results, but how efficient is it at supplying the necessary amino acids? Nitrogen is the chief ingredient of amino acids. If the bloodstream runs out of amino acids (because of insufficient protein intake), the body is said to be in nitrogen debt, or "negative nitrogen balance". Once the body builds up a nitrogen debt, there's no more tissue replacement, no more muscle growth – everything comes to a screeching halt.

Research has compared various sources in their ability to maintain positive nitrogen balance. Expressed in grams/kg of bodyweight, they stack up as follows:

Fish	.55
50:50 soy protein: fish mixture	.59
Milk	.64
50:50 soy protein: beef mixture	.66
Beef	.72
Soy protein	.75

The studies show fish as the most efficient amino acid delivery source (to maintain a positive nitrogen balance), with a fish-soy protein mixture second. Keep in mind that soy protein is virtually always used as an additive to other protein sources.

Protein powders made from milk and eggs, or milk and soy protein isolates can be mixed quickly in a blender to provide your body with a shot of high-quality protein before, between, or instead of meals occasionally. Mix as directed with milk, 1 or 2 raw eggs, and add bananas or other fruit if you prefer your milkshakes flavored.

Commit to memory that the body can only digest and assimilate about 20-30 grams of protein at one feeding, so any amount in excess of this just goes into the lake. This is yet another reason not to overeat at any one sitting. Read the labels on the protein canisters, and weigh your foods with a small kitchen scale (they only cost about $5) until you learn just how much you should consume at any one time. You get to do this 5-6 times per day, so you won't ever feel really hungry.

REMEMBER: it's not how <u>much</u> protein you eat; it's how much is <u>digested and used</u> by your body, which determines ultimate results.

The sooner you get serious about your diet, the faster your workout exercises will develop the physique you desire!

Carbohydrate Supplements

These products come in pre-bottled form or in powders that you mix yourself at home. They function strictly as a source of (almost) immediate energy. As with all purchases you make, read the labels first. If the ingredient list features glucose or dextrose and lots of preservatives, DON'T buy it. The products you <u>do</u> want to purchase, to enhance workout energy, are derived from the complex carbohydrates found in grains (maltodextrins), and this type may be a little harder to find. As described in Chapter 2, complex carbohydrates release their energy over a longer period of time than do the simple carbohydrates of sugar, thus providing you with a constant level throughout your whole workout. These products often add the electrolytes (primarily the chemical ions of sodium, potassium and magnesium) lost in sweat, as well. Gatorade is probably the best known, and the electrolytes in it help prevent muscle cramping, but they don't contain maltodextrins. I found a brand that does get its carbs from maltodextrins in a bike shop that caters to distance racers. They want this product for the same reasons YOU do, for sustained energy release over an hour or more (during your gym workouts). Buying it in bulk, in powdered form, and mixing it with water yourself is by far the least expensive way to use it. The individual bottles of pre-mixed "energy drinks" are too expensive to use on a daily basis, and they mostly contain just sugar.

Man-Made Supplements and Other Habits

In 1990, when the original version of this book was first put together, I learned about and promoted the use of many supplements to my gymnasium clientele. As a group, they are called ergogenic aids, which mean that they claim to increase performance, recuperation or otherwise enhance one's training regimen. They are made in labs, or refined from natural products (plants and herbs) in factories, and through huge advertising campaigns make the suppliers a lot of money. Everyone wants any shortcut they can find, to ripped abs and shapely muscles, no matter how far-fetched the promises are.

Twenty years later in 2012, I can't find all of those that we used back then on store shelves, but there ARE lots of others to be sure. They seem to come and go as fads.

Inosine—an ATP precursor, was hugely promoted by the Japanese, to increase the oxygen carrying capacity of the blood, to delay the onset of short-term fatigue and to delay the buildup of lactic acid in the muscles.

Octacosanol—from wheat germ oil, was touted to increase hormonal response, reaction times, aerobic efficiency and endurance, and to reduce blood pressure and heart stress—all of which are rather hard to quantify.

BCAA's—or branched-chain amino acids—particularly isoleucine, leucine and valine—are used by muscle during anaerobic work. Well, meat contains all the essential amino acids, and so do certain combinations of grains and legumes. If you'd rather eat pills than food . . . .

The list went on and on: DMG (N, N dimethyl glycine)
creatine phosphate(made from 3 amino acids)
co-enzyme Q_{10}-involved in ATP production
inositol (vitamin B_8)—as a "fat burner"
choline—with the above to aid fat metabolism
methionine—used to make creatine
MCT's—medium chain triglycerides
digestive enzymes—doubtful benefit
glandulars—processed extracts of animal glands
co-enzyme B_{12}—dibencozide from vitamin B_{12}
chromium—used to plate car bumpers etc.

OK,OK!—They probably all have a place and a use, if you've got the time and inclination to do the research before using any of them. However, I believe that mere mortals (those who just wish to slim down and get into decent beach shape, as opposed to getting into competitive posing shape) can get all the nutrition they'll ever need from good natural food.

Smoking

Does the person exist in our society who isn't aware of the reasons why one shouldn't smoke?
1. The high correlation between smoking and cancer of the lungs.
2. The high correlation between smoking and heart disease.
3. The expense (in 1990, a pack a day habit will cost you approximately $1500 per year). For those interested in the effects of inflation, 20 years later, that same habit will cost you about $3600 per year.
4. The yellow fingers, stained teeth, smelly hair and clothes.
The list could go on and on.

But here are some ways how smoking will affect your training!

1. Nicotine in cigarettes raises blood pressure and pulse rate.
2. Nicotine increases the fatty acid levels in the blood which can lead to atherosclerosis (hardening of the arteries).
3. The carbon monoxide in smoke reduces the oxygen-carrying capacity of the blood to the muscles (reduces contract-ability).
4. Smoking causes shortness of breath (bad during a heavy set).
5. Reactions to smoking in the stomach and intestines interfere with proper digestion (reducing growth potential).
6. Smoking raises your blood sugar level, thereby REDUCING your appetite.
7. Smoking shrinks capillaries and interferes with muscle growth. One puff will produce a measurable skin temperature reduction momentarily, as the capillaries constrict.

Do you need more?

Healthy people don't die in their fifties and sixties, yet almost every family has at least one dead relative who smoked, and who died young. I personally have four, a father and three uncles.

Alcohol

Alcohol is a wonderful drug that has been appreciated by countless millions in all societies throughout recorded history. It has given warriors "courage", anaesthetized patients before amputations, and made very dull parties bearable. **We** perceive it as a boon to all activities, since B.C. residents have a higher per capita consumption rate than anywhere else in Canada. Yes, we're very perceptive! But our perception is biased; we see only what we want to.

While "high" on alcohol, we find the world a relaxed and fun place to be. We sometimes get philosophical, sometimes funny. We can become amorous at inappropriate times, or with inappropriate people, and sometimes become delusional about how good we look on the dance floor. At other times, we can get depressed, moody, belligerent and/or violent. Around a drunk, you soon realize one thing. The drunk thinks he's "deep" and "attractive." You think he's stupid and boring.

Aside from the expense of all-night parties, the spousal abuse and the car accidents, what does alcohol do for your training?

Pure alcohol has NO nutritional value, but at 8 calories per gram, it is the second most concentrated source of calories, next only to pure fat (at 9 calories per gram). The higher the alcoholic content of a beverage, the more calories it contains. Alcohol is a depressant that decreases the speed of bodily functions such as thought, muscle contraction, reaction times, and digestion. Even in moderation it destroys brain cells (which are not replenished), and with heavy use destroys the liver as well. In fact, the body must devote a lot of its resources to detoxifying the bloodstream of this substance. Pop mixers—diet OR sugared—must also be detoxified.

What does this mean, **actually**??

As the body attempts to cleanse itself of the alcohol and mixers used, it flushes a tremendous amount of water (H_2O) through the kidneys—this is what accounts for the frequent trips to the bathroom, and the ensuing headaches, dizziness and stumbling around, for this water is extracted from the cells, the bloodstream and the brain. That water also carries the water-soluble minerals with it, including potassium, sodium, iron, zinc and copper. This resulting mineral imbalance is part of the "morning after" feeling, which also can include anxiety, fatigue, insomnia, depression, irritability, confusion and certainly LOW ENERGY!! A hangover is another word for "alcohol poisoning" that hasn't yet killed you.

Moderate (very moderate) use of beer, or a little wine with meals can be one of life's greatest pleasures, but heavy bouts of drinking and partying deprive you of your regular sleep pattern. You often eat incorrectly at these times, and it's easy to miss workouts when you are feeling alcohol's negative effects. So – cut way back or quit completely.

Caffeine

Coffee and tea contain no nutrients either, but both contain caffeine. Caffeine is a stimulant that increases blood pressure and speeds up bodily processes, including pulse, respiration, brain activity, and kidneys function. Too much caffeine can lead to jittery nerves, stomach irritation, and vitamin B and iron depletion. Commercial substitutes for coffee made from grains are available which contain no caffeine. Herbal teas have little or no caffeine.

Some people can't imagine beginning a day without at least one cup of coffee, and I've been one of them – "guilty as charged". And although it's pretty much a learned habit, why does it get such a hold on its devotees?

It increases the activity of the entire central nervous system (CNS). Effects noted as positives by users include: an increase in alertness and concentration, fatigue reduction, and a positive effect on strength and endurance. It is often used before training sessions for these reasons.

It has some negative effects that trainers should note:

1. It acts as a mild diuretic (makes you urinate a lot), flushing the body not only of water, but leaching calcium and electrolytes (potassium, sodium and magnesium) 3 times more than normal.
2. It increases fatty acids in the bloodstream.
3. It causes an increased risk of fibrocystic breast disease in women.
4. It increases heart rate and blood pressure, with implications for stroke and atherosclerosis.
5. It can increase irritability (which really bugs me!)

So, what's a person to do? Realize that the negative effects of caffeine may outweigh the positives, so far as your training goes. Try to limit your intake, if not eliminate it completely. Remember that there is actually NO nutrition in it that your body can use. Proper eating and good rest and sleep will leave you as alert and energetic as you need ever be, and the money you spend on coffee can be put toward more high quality protein, fruit and vegetables.

Sleep

Maximum muscle growth can only take place when the body gets sufficient sleep and rest. This means at least eight hours of sound, restful sleep each night. Since the body thrives on regularity, going to bed at the same time each evening will help because the body will be accustomed to falling asleep during certain hours. This will result in more restful slumber. After a long day and a good workout, there are many worn-out cells that need replacing. Not only does growth and repair take place during periods of sleep and rest, but sleep is necessary for mental health also. Although the sleep requirement for each individual varies somewhat, to ensure optimum muscle growth, 8-10 hours is recommended. Trainers who are serious about accomplishing their goals need more sleep than the average person, and many try to incorporate an afternoon nap into their schedule.

CHAPTER 4 Regulating Your Metabolism

All of the physical, chemical, and electrical processes that occur in the building up, activity, and breaking down of body cells are called the *metabolism*. This involves the flow of energy into and out of the cells, and the conversion of food energy into heat and motion.

The two main divisions of metabolism are: (1) ANABOLISM, the building up of tissue; maintenance and repair of the body and (2) CATABOLISM, the breaking down of tissue for energy production and excretion.

Less academically, metabolism, or metabolic rate, is the speed at which the body processes energy. You could compare it to the idle of a car. Typically, a person with a stringy, thin build has a very high or fast metabolic rate. His "engine" races at high speed; all foods consumed are burned rapidly and weight gain is nearly impossible. In the gym, he is known as a "hard gainer", and should definitely let the suggested 10% of the diet devoted to fat consumption rise to double that. The person who is slow-moving, often overweight, big-boned and placid in nature invariably has a slow metabolism. His (or her) engine idles slowly and sluggishly. It doesn't burn fuel efficiently and weight gain in the form of fat is all too easy.

In general, children have fast metabolic rates. They run around all day long (did you ever try to follow one, step for step, for more than a few minutes?), eat anything and everything, and never gain an ounce. As a person ages, the metabolic rate gradually slows; we often become less active, and sometimes gain fat while barely eating anything. There is definitely a major shift in the way our bodies metabolize food, which occurs around the age of 30. What you could eat and drink at ages younger than this has an entirely different effect on your body as you age – UNLESS you control your metabolism, and this is not only possible, but required, if you want a slim, fit healthy body. Even if you are 30-ish, slim and/or fit, any poor eating habits that have seemed to "work" so far won't for long. Learn the information in this book and try to practice it from now on.

What is the ideal state of metabolism for a bodybuilder? Obviously, a fast metabolism is no good – you can't gain shapely muscular weight. A slow metabolism is equally unwanted. You will continue to look "shapeless" despite lots of well-intentioned gym work. The condition you want is a healthy, vigorous NORMAL metabolic rate. If you already have one, you are lucky indeed. Your training will produce maximal results right from the start.

Fast Metabolisms Must Be Slowed Down

A super-fast metabolism is the enemy of the skinny bodybuilder. Most are in total despair. They eat and drink huge quantities of the "right" foods, yet they fail to gain more than a pound or two of muscle per year. These people, known as ectomorphs, are easy to recognize. They are often tall and gangly, with no fat on their bodies. Also, they usually have no visible muscular development either. A person with a fast metabolic rate is often worrying about something, and usually cannot relax either physically or mentally.

How can the fast metabolism be corrected? The obvious answer is immobilization. You should be as lazy as your lifestyle will permit. It's far better to take a desk job than to do manual labor. You should train intensely, using 30-40 minute routines, rather than to train for the more normal 1-1½ hours; and you should (temporarily, at least) limit other physical sports and pastimes.

You must purposely practice relaxation. Relax during the day, particularly for 30 minutes after meals or your between-meal protein shakes or other nutritious snack, to help facilitate proper digestion and assimilation of nutrients. Never do anything physical immediately after eating. Remember Mom's hated rule? – You can't go swimming for at least 45 minutes after lunch, or you'll get cramps and die! She may have been a little overboard there, but certainly was "on the right track". Why? Because the blood supply necessary to help digestion will be mainly in your gut area after eating, and not so much in the muscles which might tend to cramp up without it.

Mental stress is just as detrimental to a fast metabolism as physical stress. It is usually self-imposed. You worry about things over which you have no control and you must learn that the choice to worry is yours alone to make. Do you like being tense? Of course not, but what can you DO about it? At times like these I have found that the best way to counteract such feelings is with some form of physical exertion. If it's time for a workout, great! Go pump some iron. But if not, go rake the lawn, walk your dog, dig up the garden . . . You WILL calm down. Be honest with yourself and choose to believe that the world is going to "unfold" before you, naturally, whether you worry, or not. Relax . . . breathe deeply, and slowly. Rid yourself of tension and unwanted physical and mental stress. Just as you can control your body's shape with proper exercise and nutrition, you can control your mental state with practice and self-confidence. You, and only you, are in charge of your life.

In the gym, the ectomorph with a fast metabolism has amazing recuperative powers, and there is a need for frequent, relatively short workouts 5 or even 6 times per week, at around 85% intensity. Keep the number of repetitions per set to 6-8. Training to the limit (100% intensity) all the time stops gains dead; the system is always overburdened. The hard gainer should do very little or **NO ABDOMINAL WORK**, since this area is easily traumatized, which means that you can work it to the extent that it will signal the rest of the body to stop growing.

The hard gainer needs variety, both in nutrition and exercise. You should change your routine frequently, every few weeks, but be careful not to over train by adding exercises to an existing routine. Keep your routine short, and hard. Keep amino acids high in the blood by eating small, regular quantities of high-protein foods, such as meat, fish, milk and eggs. Take a good quality milk-and-egg protein supplement between meals for positive nitrogen balance. This will provide a never-ending source of muscle-building fuel so that your blood sugar never drops.

The slim body will add shapely muscular mass, and as the fast metabolism slows down to a "normal" rate, bodyweight will rise. The ectomorph gradually becomes a mesomorph, the traditionally coveted athletic physique, the one with lots of muscle while retaining the low body fat percentage they began with.

Slow Metabolisms Must Be Sped Up

How? By activity and by diet.

I stated in the introduction that severe dieting to lose weight can slow the metabolism by up to 45%. I hope we've already agreed that any sort of "crash" or fad diet is NOT the way to go, and that a moderate approach to your goal will serve you better over time. If you've "tried every diet in the book", you know that NONE of them work for long. Sorry, it will take a lifestyle change to CHANGE YOU.

Aerobics (much more on this in Chapter 9) can be used to energize the system, and normalize your body's chemical processes. After embracing and beginning this stimulating work, your digestive system will accelerate; your glands will secrete more; your hormones will be stirred up. In all the gym exercises you do, the overweight (over fat) trainer should use light weights and do high repetitions in order to burn off as much body fat as possible and at the same time build shapely muscles.

If you are more than 50 pounds "over fat" (clinically obese) you are going to have to have patience, and a strong belief in the methods presented here. The task may seem almost too awesome to begin – but the options to beginning, have even worse long-term effects. You already believe this, or you wouldn't now be reading. The person who has gotten badly "out-of-shape" must remember that conditions that have taken years to achieve, will take a full year to reverse – and that doing this, is worth it.

Reversing the Muscle-Loss/Fat-Gain Spiral

Being quite overweight is not always so much the fault of a sluggish metabolism, as it is the result of a sedentary lifestyle coupled with poor eating habits, but these two are very closely related. The body doesn't burn off many calories, and packs on excess food intake very easily as fat. Everyone with a sedentary lifestyle will lose approximately 10% of their body's lean muscle mass per decade after the age of 20, and in general it will be replaced by fat. It is important to note that:

ENERGY STORED IN EXCESS FAT CELLS IS BURNED <u>ONLY</u> IN MUSCLE CELLS

So—if we <u>allow</u> ourselves to lose muscle mass through inactivity as we age, we decrease our ability to burn fat away, and thus increase the likelihood of gaining weight in the form of more fat. This muscle-loss/fat-gain "spiral" is the prime cause of obesity (along with over eating the wrong kinds of food).

To reverse this process, it will be necessary to make the huge commitment to a <u>lifestyle change</u>. The inactive person must become more active and start eating the correct foods and supplements in the correct quantities.

<u>The Walking Program</u>

To enhance the muscle to fat ratio, it will be necessary to train 3 times per week with bodybuilding exercises (to create muscle tissue), and on alternate days to follow a program of walking, to begin the fat loss process. The weight training will be relatively easy because the overweight individual doesn't have to move very much, but depending on how far you've "let things go", walking 100 meters (roughly the distance between 2 telephone poles, or perhaps a city block) may seem like miles. Every "walking" day, walk further until you can walk for 60 minutes. However far you go, keep an eye on your watch, note where you are at 10 minutes "out" say, then head for home. You will have walked for 20 minutes. Keep raising the time you walk by going further than the last session – pass the previous point where you turned around by 100 or 200 meters, and head back. For 20 minutes "out" you'll get a total walking time of 40 minutes. THAT is improvement you can be proud of. Work your way up over a few weeks so that you can walk a 60 minute return trip home. At that point, try walking progressively faster, so that you can cover greater distances in the same 60 minutes (you needn't walk for more than an hour – there are other things to do in this life!). If you have access to a 400m track, you can easily note the number of laps you can complete, yet still be near your car. This part of your training will burn off calories, and therefore fat; you will have more energy daily as you carry around a body that is getting slightly smaller every day, and as you build your strength and lean muscle mass in the gym on alternate days, your metabolic rate will begin to rise. <u>The increasing muscle mass will make it easier to burn ever more fat.</u> In short, your metabolism will start to normalize – you are beginning to **reverse** the spiral toward obesity and back toward a slimmer, stronger body. Be proud of yourself – pat yourself on the back – this is starting to work!!

Eating the correct foods will also help balance a slow metabolism. Junk foods such as sugary soft drinks, cookies and "refined" products will ultimately <u>slow down</u> the metabolic rate, whereas fresh eggs, vegetables, seafood, and fruits will serve to speed it up. Eat NOTHING with flour or sugar in it! Eat less (read "NO") processed foods. Higher protein intake will <u>increase</u> your metabolic rate up to 30%.

Once you have normalized your metabolism, the bulky "endomorphic" body will, like the slim "ectomorph", begin to become the desired "mesomorphic" type – lots of shapely muscle and energy, and a low body fat percentage. By adopting proper eating habits and accepting that training for muscularity and other physical activities must become a <u>lifelong</u> habit, it is likely that you will never again have a very fast OR a very slow metabolic rate. If there is some change, however, it is usually evidenced by a <u>slowing</u> down of the metabolism as you age.

If you feel that your system is getting sluggish, you can again take steps to hype it with more aerobic activities such as bike riding and swimming. Aerobic activity can speed up your metabolic rate by as much as 25% for 15 hours after you finish exercising. It also tends to depress the appetite. Add to this the calories used in performing the exercise, and you can see the value of aerobic activity combined with a sensible eating plan for fat reduction. See Chapter 9.

CHAPTER 5 Eating For Function

Whatever your reasons may be, you go to a gym because you want to change the shape of your body – and you are not alone. The bulky people want to be smaller; the skinny ones want to be bigger. There are people in the gym who look "normal" in clothes, being neither overweight nor underweight, but who are soft and weak. They want to get stronger and leaner.

All three types and everyone in between, need to eat foods favorable to lean muscle mass increase, and to limit (or eliminate completely) those foods conducive to gaining fat. In other words, you must begin to

EAT FOR FUNCTION, NOT FOR FUN

Whenever you are about to put something in your mouth, you should ask yourself "Is this going to help or hinder me in my quest for my ideal body?" Why would you eat or drink anything that doesn't contribute to your goal? A "Slurpy" isn't food, you know!

Eating for function, the bodybuilder's way, requires that a few concepts be reviewed, before going on.

First, the body needs energy (calories). It also needs vitamins, minerals, and enzymes. Complex carbohydrate foods contain vitamins, minerals and enzymes as well as calories, at the rate of four calories per gram. Some fats contain some vitamins, but they are concentrated sources of calories also, at nine calories per gram. This is a bad trade-off, and so, fats should be eliminated. Processed carbohydrates also provide energy at four calories per gram, but generally contain no nutrients; therefore, they too, should be eliminated. We need high quality protein in the amounts of approximately 1-2 grams per kilogram of bodyweight, spread over 5-6 small meals per day. Protein also supplies energy calories, at four calories per gram.

You will have to remember, and apply, the following rule when choosing foods to consume.

Feed Your Muscles – Starve Your Fat

We must eat foods that give us the greatest return in nutrients for each calorie they provide, while at the same time resisting those foods that can only make us fatter; the ones that provide "empty" calories (no nutrients).

At first, the bodybuilder's diet may seem rather bland and uninteresting, but as you start to see the results materializing, this will seem less and less of a problem. Also, your tastes will change. Food that is over-salted, over-sugared, and "processed" will become more and more distasteful to you – your body's way of telling you that it is unnatural and unhealthy food for you.

Eat to live; **DON'T** live to eat!

In your choice of foods, THINK "nutrition first". Cut out all processed and junk foods from your diet. Remember that a "Twinkies and coffee" diet will produce a "Twinkies and coffee" body! If you have a choice between a baked potato and greasy (oil-soaked) French fries, take the baked potato. Fresh fruits and vegetables are better than canned; raw is better than steamed; steamed (lightly) is better than boiled. Stone-ground whole-wheat bread is better than "refined" white bread (mechanical high-temperature grinding destroys enzymes). A glass of skim milk (0% fat) is better for you than 1%(fat) milk; 1%(fat) milk is better than 2%(fat) milk, and 2%(fat) milk is better than homogenized (3.5%fat) milk – but one glass of any of the four would have more nutrition in it and do more for your physique than a whole <u>case</u> of soda pop, diet or sugared. NO nutrition there, at all!

Try and eat as many raw or lightly cooked foods as possible. Thus vital nutrients and enzymes are not destroyed in the cooking process, and the foods are easier to digest. For example, almost raw meat (steak "tartar") digests in your stomach in one hour, while "well-done" meats take over four hours, burdening your system.

This doesn't mean you can never indulge yourself a little. Most top-flight bodybuilders have what they call their "junk food day" to help them get through their Spartan pre-contest diets. Although I personally do not recommend junk food, I think you should satisfy a craving occasionally and have that pizza (not a whole one!), ice cream, beer, chocolate bar, or whatever your particular thing is. Everyone's got one – mine is salty snacks. Trust your body's wisdom that you <u>need</u> a bit of that "food" which is not normally part of your nutritional plan, and indulge in whatever you crave. Just keep your ultimate goal of the slim strong body in mind, and limit your indulgence to no more than once a week, and watch the quantity. Remember the super-models' motto:

Nothing tastes as good as being slim feels!

Practical Ways to Cut Fat Intake

It is not necessary to <u>ever</u> feel deprived of food <u>volume</u> while on a bodybuilding diet. By cutting down the number of calories ingested that come from fat, you can eat far <u>more</u> of the nutritious foods that contain the vitamins, minerals and enzymes required by your body.

Standing in supermarket lines, I can't help observing other people's food choices. The "bulkier" a person is, the more likely their shopping cart is to contain canned and packaged foods, high fat cuts of meat, salad dressings, cookies and Cheezies (Yum!—dang). They will have white bread, butter and processed cheese slices—<u>all</u> high-calorie, nutrient-poor foods. The unfortunate thing is that they probably think that they are eating correctly for health. Their children are being "set up" for nutritional failure (obesity).

Restaurant patrons typically avoid the "starchy" foods, such as potatoes and bread, while putting scoops of dressing on their salad. Or they "ration" themselves to one-half a roll but use two pats of butter on it. They don't seem to realize that an entire baked potato contains fewer calories than two tablespoons of salad dressing. The cautious bread eater would be calorically wiser if he ate <u>two</u> whole rolls and <u>omitted</u> the butter. Moreover, it should be evident to everyone by now, that the vitamins, minerals and fiber are in the rolls and potato, not the butter, sour cream or salad dressing.

Why do people so often say that carbohydrates are fattening? **FAT IS FATTENING!** By cutting out fat, you can eat as much as, or more than usual, and yet reduce calorie consumption by 40 to 50 percent. That means a progressively slimmer you.

What follows, are ways to eliminate fat from each of the food groups.

Cutting Fat from the Milk Group

One glass of whole (homogenized) milk is the same as one glass of skim milk—with two pats of butter added. Actually, skim milk has a slightly higher percentage of protein than homogenized milk because the fat removed from the 3.5% fat milk is replaced by even more skim milk. The word "homogenized" merely means that the fat in the milk is so well distributed that it will not float on top, as in farmer's whole milk. You can slowly wean yourself from homogenized milk to skim milk by starting to buy the 2% (fat) version for a week or two, then move to 1% (fat) milk for a while, and finally on to skim milk, gradually becoming used to the less-fattening taste. You will soon get used to the more watery texture of the skim. All the nutrients are still there, but the fat is gone. You will likely be consuming a lot of protein shakes, and you will need the skim milk as mixer.

If you're a yogurt-lover, apply the same theory. Read the labels and then take the low-fat or non-fat brands. The fruit-flavored kinds may be low in fat, but are high in sugars so limit your amounts of these. Plain non-fat yogurt can be used as a base for salad dressings, vegetable toppings, and makes a reasonably good substitute for sour cream on your baked potato.

Although its name implies the contrary, buttermilk is very low in fat (1.5%fat). One cup contains 140 calories, which come from 11g of protein (44 calories), 4g of fat (36 calories), and 15g of carbs (60 calories).You can make a tasty low-fat snack by blending it with a little frozen fruit concentrate (watch out for the high sugar content here) or fresh fruits like strawberries or blueberries. Many baking recipes that call for whole milk will yield more flavorful and less fattening results when you substitute buttermilk, but in general, try to resist baked goods. It also comes in a "light" version. One cup has 8g of protein, 2g of fat, 12g of carbs, and tastes almost exactly the same.

Cheese is a favorite food for millions of people, but unfortunately it is a super concentrated source of calories. When producers brag that it takes 20 glasses of milk to make a small brick of cheese, they are really saying that as the water is removed from the milk, the fat in it is progressively concentrated, making it one of the worst things you can eat, in terms of your bodybuilding goals. If you really cannot resist, at least try to follow these suggestions:

1. Cheese is white, not orange. Avoid the chemically colored cheeses. Your body doesn't need to detoxify "the unpronounceable additives".
2. Read the labels, and choose the ones with the lowest percentage fat content.
3. Use the old or "nippy" versions, not the mild or medium ones. You can use much less and still get plenty of cheesy taste.
4. Cottage cheese is fine, and comes in low-fat or non-fat labeled containers. Choose these, instead of the full-fat "creamed" ones.
5. Lastly, eat less cheese than you would normally.

While on the subject of "creamed" products, eliminate them completely from your menu. This means creamy salad dressings, creamy soups, ice cream, and cream in your tea or coffee. You might as well swallow I0-W-30 – it's all pure added fat.

Cutting Fat from the Meat Group

Trim the fat off everything! And cut the fat off before you cook. This applies to chicken as well as beef. If you remove the skin from a whole chicken before cooking you'll eliminate about 55% of the calories. If you wait until after cooking to remove the skin, then some of the fat under the skin stays on the meat and you'll cut only about half as many calories.

When cooking ground beef in a skillet, elevate one side of the skillet on a spoon and brown the meat on the elevated side, allowing the fat to drain down to the low side. You can spoon it out for disposal this way without allowing it to soak into the meat. Again, read labels here. Buy "extra lean " before "lean." Never buy "regular" ground beef—it's too fatty.

When cooking meats, the method is important. Frying in pans usually involves the addition of oil or butter first, so frying should be avoided. Roast, broil or BBQ your meat. Better yet, use a wok– you don't need oil in a wok; water or bouillon will do the job just as well.

If you love red meat, stick to the lower-fat cuts such as flank and round steak. They have the added advantage of being cheaper than their high fat cousins—tenderloin and T bone steaks, and prime rib roasts. We pay extra for fat. Internalize **that!**

Top-flight physiques seldom (if ever) eat pork (including ham and bacon), lamb, or veal. The percentage of fat in them is just too high. The same is true of hot dogs, bologna, and most pre-formed, sliced luncheon meats. Like canned meat and sausages, smoked and "cured" meats are all heavily laced with chemical preservatives to keep their high fat content from becoming rancid. You don't need any of these products. Don't buy them at all. EVER!

White fleshed fish is a good high-protein low-fat bargain. Just like the 2 types of meat on poultry (chicken and turkey), white fleshed fish are leaner than their dark meat relatives. Chicken breast (white meat) is less fatty than chicken thigh and leg (dark meat). White fish like cod, halibut, sole and flounder are less fatty than pink salmon, trout and char. As with poultry, skin fish before cooking if possible and don't fry them in oil or butter. Broil, barbecue or poach them lightly. If you buy canned tuna, get it "water packed", not packed in oil. And remember to rinse the salt off before consuming it.

Cutting Fat from the Fruit and Vegetable Group

Most fruits and vegetables are nutritious, low-fat, high-fiber foods and they should comprise a large part of your daily intake, to provide much-needed energy, vitamins, and minerals. Their value is impaired by many people when they add gobs of greasy dressings or sugary syrups and toppings. Flavorful low-fat toppings are easy to make on your own. Experiment with mixtures of low-fat yogurt, spices, wine, lemon juice, bouillon, and other seasonings (but <u>not</u> salt).

There are several tricks whereby you can have your salad dressing without the high calories. You can mix it with half a glass of milk, producing a "calorie-reduced" dressing. In restaurants, you can order oil and vinegar, or lemon juice to be brought to you "on the side", so that you can add as <u>little</u> oil as you wish.

With the exception of avocados and olives, fruits and vegetables are low in fats. Again, learn how to top them with creative low-fat sauces rather than butter, cream sauces, or cheese. A baked potato is great topped with a blend of cottage cheese, chives, mustard, and Worcestershire sauce.

People should eat the natural whole fruit or vegetable, rather than juicing or drying it. A whole apricot has more fiber and fewer free sugars than a glass of apricot juice. A handful of raisins has the sugar from a small basket full of grapes concentrated into a mouthful – definitely too many calories, if you have many (handfuls, that is!).

Cutting Fat from the Bread and Cereal Group

Just because bread is dark in color doesn't mean it's high in fiber. When I say "read the label", I am referring to the list of ingredients—not the title on the package. If it doesn't say 100% whole wheat or whole rye then it isn't "the right stuff". The more whole grain a product contains, the higher its fiber content, and if the fiber content is high, the calories will be low, because the fiber tends to be difficult to digest and "ties up" many of the calories. They are (then) not digested, and go right through you.

High-fiber cereals such as shredded wheat and bran, topped with fruit and skim milk make a great breakfast. If you buy packaged cereals, read the labels. If sugar is in the list, don't buy it. Your body doesn't need it.

In baking (if you <u>must</u> do it) you can safely cut the oil and sugar in a recipe by at least half without spoiling the flavor. Another way to cut fat in baked goods is to use two egg whites and one yolk when a recipe calls for two whole eggs. Save the yolks for your between-meal protein shakes. You can also substitute low-fat or skim milk for whole milk.

While you can control what you eat at home quite easily, restaurant eating can pose difficulties. Try to order all dishes "dry"; that is, no mayonnaise (60% fat) or butter (100% fat) on toast or sandwiches, no sauces on the entrées, no dressings on the salads. Ask the waiter to bring condiments on the side so you can control quantities. Avoid menu items described as "dipped in batter", "fried", "creamed", or "in a sauce". If you order alcoholic drinks, add water, club soda, or diet soda to your wine or liquor.

10 ways to Drop 5 Pounds

1. Eat breakfast. If you don't feel up to <u>solid</u> food in the morning, make a high-protein, nutritious "shake" to help "break your fast". Add two tablespoons of a high-quality milk-and-egg protein powder, ten ounces of skim milk, and a banana or other fruit for flavor. Add a raw egg or two for even more protein.

2. Skip the "mayo" on your sandwich and save yourself 50-100 calories. Gradually reduce from butter on both sides, to only one side, to "dry". Add a little mustard or ketchup (low in fat) if you need the moisture. Try turkey or chicken instead of pastrami, ham or cheese.

3. Park a few blocks from where you work. The walk will invigorate you mentally and physically, as well as burning a few calories. And take the stairs whenever you can—elevators don't burn a thing except electricity.

4. Clean the kitchen—not the cabinet doors etc.—clean out **the fridge**. Dump all the high-fat cheeses, desserts,

cream, whole milk, and high-calorie dressings. If they're not there, you can't eat them.

5. Enjoy your dinner by eating more slowly, slower than feels natural. It takes about 20 minutes for the brain to get the message that your blood sugar level has risen. If you eat too fast, you consume more than necessary, because your brain doesn't know you are "full" yet.

6. Soup is like water, it helps to fill you up. Have broth before dinner so you will eat less of the main dish.

7. Skip the chips and dip at parties. Stick to <u>unbuttered</u> popcorn, while avoiding the <u>salted</u> nuts and pretzels. Take your own if you wish (or if you must).

8. Walk around at work. Take the mail out yourself. Do your own photocopying, carry a memo to a colleague, and get your own coffee.

9. Get rid of the snacks in your desk. On breaks, pull out fruit or vegetable sticks from home. Jelly doughnuts have a way of making you resemble them.

10. And if you can manage it, "get lucky" before breakfast. It'll burn about 100 calories (depending on various factors) and get your mind off food.

Try these suggestions for a few weeks and see how all the little things can "add up" to subtract the pounds.

HOW BADLY DO YOU WANT THE LEAN PHYSIQUE?

Enough to follow some, or all, of this book's suggestions, I hope!

CHAPTER 6 When Should You Eat?

The Metabolic Needs Curve

The following chart is meant to illustrate a very important principle. We have previously explained that calories are not only ingested (as food), but are expended (through activity). On the chart below are 2 lines – the solid one roughly approximates the general caloric needs of a person who has a day job. After awakening sometime before 8AM, we should be feeding ourselves so as to enable us to dress and get ready for whatever work or play we wish to engage in.

This feeding should "get us through" until the next one (usually around noon), at which time we will be replenishing our cells and muscles, and to provide energy in **advance** for the rest of the afternoon. You can see that while our caloric needs are relatively low <u>first thing</u> in the morning, we need a substantial breakfast to power our morning's activities. Our needs peak around noon, so we need plenty of intake around that time as well. As we use up this lunchtime nutrition and go through the afternoon, our needs drop, and so our evening meal around 6PM should be quite small; we usually don't do too much strenuous activity after that, and we are "winding down" toward bedtime, when our caloric needs drop to almost zero for sleeping.

Unfortunately, many people don't match their caloric intake with their actual needs, thus giving rise to the second (dotted) line on the chart. They often have little or no breakfast, grab a small lunch somewhere along the way, have a big dinner (around 6PM), then snack until bedtime.

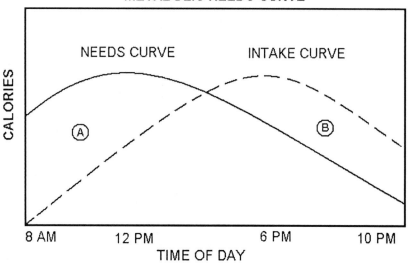

METABOLIC NEEDS CURVE

NEEDS CURVE   INTAKE CURVE

CALORIES

Ⓐ   Ⓑ

8 AM   12 PM   6 PM   10 PM

TIME OF DAY

Look at the chart above, again. The area labeled "A" between the solid and the dotted line indicates a morning and afternoon wherein our needs exceed our intake. We may feel weak, lethargic, irritable, and prone to headaches . . . , and all because we haven't fed our muscle and brain cells sufficiently, and on-time, to enable them to perform their required tasks optimally.

Now look at the area labeled "B". Now we're in the late afternoon/ evening period. We're HUNGRY, due to insufficient intake during our workday. We have a big meal, relax, maybe a drink or two to "unwind", certainly are not entertaining any thoughts of going to the gym or out for a bike ride . . . maybe watch a little TV, a few more snacks. Since our energy output (need) is very low, but our caloric intake is high, the difference is stored as . . . You guessed it, FAT!!

Now, here is the good news. Look at the peak on both curves – without getting overly technical, our intake should about match our needs at any given time, in order to neither gain nor lose weight. To lose weight, your total daily intake must be less than your output, and to gain weight you must take in more calories than you expend. Since you already know WHAT foods you should be eating, it's now just a question of WHEN you should ingest the required nutrition, and how much of it you should have at each feeding.

WE MUST ALIGN THESE TWO CURVES!!

It has been said that breakfast is the most important meal of the day, for it fuels the first few hours. You really owe it to yourself to be as alert and cheerful around your family, friends and co-workers as possible and great nutrition makes this possible. Make your breakfast large and nutritious. Mid-morning, have a smallish carb/protein snack. Your caloric needs remain high, so make your lunch pretty substantial as well. Since you need to work all afternoon, and perhaps hit the gym for a workout, or go for some cardiovascular activity (a run, walk, bike ride . . . .) afterwards, you should be planning in a small nutritious snack about an hour or so before that activity. A smallish supper is all you need as your energy requirements lessen throughout the evening, and a small amount digesting in your stomach makes for a more restful sleep. That means you get to eat 5 times per day, and if the makeup of these meals is correct, you will never get very hungry, if at all. In fact, you MAY have to remind yourself to eat at your preplanned times. Keep before bedtime snacking to a minimum. You will then wake up fairly hungry, want to have that solid nourishing breakfast, and keep this programmed meal timing going.

There is an old expression: Eat breakfast like a King, lunch like a Prince, and dinner like a pauper. Apparently they knew about the metabolic needs curve back in the 1600's.

The preceding information has been VERY general, and will suffice for most people, but if you wish to get into it a little deeper, and have a few of the concepts mentioned previously "fleshed out" a bit, read on.

It has been stated that it would be best for a person to "graze" all day long, but for most this is impossible. Our society has made a big deal out of eating "three square meals" per day, and most people badly abuse even this advice, as the metabolic needs curve above explains. The ideal way for trainers to eat for fat loss and muscular development is 5-6 small meals per day. Let's go with 5 feedings (unless you are a competition bodybuilder – then you get 6!), spaced about 3 hours apart. In order of importance, here's the lineup:

1. the pre-workout meal – about 1½-2 hours before
2. the post-workout meal – (in 2 parts) – carbohydrates **alone** about 30 minutes after, then protein **alone** about an hour after
3. breakfast—this becomes #1 if you wish to train early in the day
4. & 5 – these other 2 meals fit in around the first 3

What Should Comprise These Meals?

I always try to work from the general to the specific, so if the first three suggestions below are all you wish to master at this point, FINE!!

I will then explain something called the glycemic index, and proceed with a more in-depth way of calculating your protein requirements. This part will probably appeal more to trainers with competitive desires, than for "more normal folk"!

How much should I eat? Follow the two-fist rule

Look at your hands, put your two fists together, and **that volume** is "roughly" the size your stomach **should be**, even if you've distended it through over-indulgence. Therefore, your plate shouldn't have more on it, IN TOTAL, than the combined volume of your two fists! If you are used to eating quite a lot more than that, don't worry, your stomach will soon regain its normal size. Also, you are going to get this amount every 3 hours or so, so you probably won't ever feel really hungry, at all.

What should be on my plate? Follow the 2/3:1/3 rule

Two thirds of your smallish plate (see rule #1 above) should have your carbohydrate portion on it, and the remaining one third should be your protein. None of this "steak hanging over both sides, and a spoonful of salad" stuff. Now, some foods contain BOTH carbohydrates and protein, as noted in Chapter 2.

Make it colorful! The 2/3 of the plate that is carbohydrates.

Yes, that will ensure that you get some red tomatoes, green or yellow or leafy vegetables, orange or red or green peppers, turnip, radishes, green onions, brown rice, white buckwheat, red kidney beans . . . . you get it!!! You can go back and look at the chart near the end of Chapter 2 to refresh your mind as to how important the vegetables are. That's where most of our vitamins, minerals and enzymes come from.

Let's Go Deeper—The Glycemic Index

Carbs are your primary source for energy-giving muscle glycogen. Of course, fats and proteins can also contribute to energy for sustained workouts, but 85% of your muscle glycogen should come from carbs. Carbohydrates are not all equal in the rate at which they are converted to blood glucose and (ultimately) muscle glycogen. Because of this, some foods from each category are superior in their ability to yield long-term energy. Simple sugars are converted to blood glucose (the "refined" fuel) very rapidly. Bodybuilders know they should shy away from such simple carbs because, while blood glucose rises sharply, it also falls rapidly and your energy hits the rocks. It's not all that simple, though. Carbohydrates are rated according to a formula known as the glycemic index. Most simple sugars have a glycemic index that's very high; that is, they are converted to glucose very rapidly. Glucose, in fact, is given the glycemic index of 100, and is the basis against which all other foods are judged. When you become used to reading the labels on foods you buy, you will likely be astounded at how often glucose heads the list. Ingredients on labels are listed from highest % to lowest %, so whatever is first and second on the list will be your tip-off.

Well, the simple sugar called fructose (the natural form of sugar found in fruits) has a glycemic index of only 20! That's right, 20! It is an excellent pre-workout source of carbohydrates because it keeps your blood glucose levels relatively stable for a long period of time.

Conversely, potatoes, typically thought of as a good source of energy, have a glycemic index of 90! Bad pre-workout food! There are many surprises on the accompanying table of glycemic indexes of foods. Foods once considered excellent energy foods really aren't, and other foods you may have disregarded show up as vital to your long-term energy levels.

Study the table below:

100%	glucose
80-90%	corn flakes, carrots, parsnips, potatoes, maltose, and honey
70-79%	whole wheat bread, millet, white rice, Weetabix, fresh broad beans, new potatoes
60-69%	white bread, brown rice, muesli, shredded wheat, Ryvita biscuits, beets, bananas, raisins, Mars bar
50-59%	buckwheat, white spaghetti, sweet corn, All-bran, digestive biscuits, frozen peas, yams, sucrose (table sugar), potato chips
40-49%	whole wheat spaghetti, oatmeal porridge, sweet potato, canned navy beans, dried peas, oranges, orange juice
30-39%	butter beans, haricot beans, black eye peas, chick peas, apples (golden delicious), ice cream, skim milk, whole milk, yogurt, tomato soup
20-29%	kidney beans, lentils, fructose (fruit sugar)
10-19%	soy beans (whole or canned), peanuts (but really high in fat!)

Your Carbohydrate Intake Objectives

1) Your pre-workout meal should be eaten about 2 hours before training – low (or no) fat, high in protein (but<30g), medium complex carbs (~50 grams) – mainly low glycemic index, (beans and fruit—except bananas, are best). The carbs needed during your workout come mainly from the meal eaten 5-8 hours previously. This would be your breakfast or mid-morning feeding if you train in the late afternoon.

About an hour later, and before you begin your workout, start sipping your maltodextrin carb drink (mentioned in the supplement section). Make it last at least halfway through your training session. Not only do you want to get through your workout with plenty of energy for the sets you must do to excel, but you must also have plenty of energy reserves to replace those spent during the workout. For about 45-60 minutes following your training session, your muscles are busy restoring energy and removing catabolic waste materials in preparation for the anabolic process (muscle-building phase) that follows. You can have a small carb feeding about ½ hour after training to facilitate the replenishment of this energy (high glycemic index carbs are OK here, for quick absorption). Anabolism will be incomplete if the first stage is incomplete. Furthermore, if you have little or no reserves of energy, your muscles will be cannibalized for the necessary energy to replace that spent during the workout.

2) Your post-workout meal should be consumed about one hour after you are finished training. That's about when energy stores have been replenished and anabolism begins. You need this meal to be high in protein, since the most rapid amino acid uptake occurs 90-120 minutes after your training session, and protein you've eaten 60 minutes after your workout will be already partially digested, absorbed through the villi (the actual site of absorption) in your intestines and available in the bloodstream during this time "window of opportunity" interval.

3) Every meal during the day should have a good mix of carbohydrates. Aside from your post-workout meal, the others (at least 4) should have plenty of carbs with a range of glycemic indexes. If all you ingest are high glycemic index carbs, your blood sugar will soar and then drop precipitously, causing your energy to crash long before your next meal. Some of these meals or snacks should

contain raw or lightly steamed vegetables, and/or raw fruit, which provide not only vitamins and minerals, but also indigestible fiber which improves elimination of solid wastes.

4) On days you don't train, reduce your caloric intake accordingly, but stick to a good mix of carbs as above. On low activity days, you don't need as much energy, so don't take in as much food because whatever you don't use is stored as fat. Once stored, fat tends to stay stored. This fat is NOT reclaimed as energy the next day, but instead your energy comes from your food the next day, plus (if you've goofed in your estimation of how much to eat at each meal and take in too little) cannibalized muscle tissue – that's the same muscle tissue you work so hard to build! Energy needs beyond your caloric intake are NOT readily available from reclaimed fat stores. THAT takes aerobic training – see Chapter 7.

We have been talking as if carbs were all you need to eat, and that they should be all raw vegetables, and I think some clarification is needed. We also know that we need protein, and tend to think it must all come from animal sources. This too, is an over simplification. Many carbohydrate sources are also excellent sources of protein if combined properly to yield *complete* protein, as was explained way back in Chapter 2. Fat hides almost everywhere (as was shown in Chapter 5) so we don't have to look for sources of what little need we have for fat. We also know that the amount of protein we need depends on our activity level, and on our size. Obviously a large champion bodybuilder has greater protein needs than an office worker who wants to do a little gym training to get in shape for jogging, tennis and dancing. If we can determine your protein needs (in grams per feeding), then we can pick our sources to suit our individual tastes, and decide how much of each one to eat by careful label reading before making up our plates.

Calculating Your Lean Bodyweight

Dr. Fred Hatfield (nicknamed Dr. Squat in the power lifting world, the first man to ever squat with 1000 pounds!, and an actual PhD in the social sciences of sport as well) has developed the following procedure for determining daily protein requirements, based upon lean body weight and activity level. He has been an instructor of mine, and has given me permission to duplicate the following charts. You can consult them to roughly determine your daily protein requirements, but to use the second one we first need to determine what is known as your "Lean Bodyweight". This is for the following reason, stated two ways.

1) The portion of your total weight that is **fat** has 0 protein requirements. It's just along for the ride.
2) Fat is only "burned" in muscles, so it is only your lean bodyweight that has protein needs.

There are body composition tests you can have done to determine your Lean Bodyweight (LBW), but they cost money, and you need access to some pretty high-tech facilities and equipment. The following examples should help you find yourself on the charts which follow.

If you are an in-shape, pre-contest bodybuilder, you probably have VERY little body fat, your muscles are very visible, and striations show when you flex. Your body fat % is in the 5% range, and your LBW is therefore ~95% of your total weight. If you weigh 220 pounds, your LBW is 95% x 220 = 209 pounds. Approximately 4% of your body's fat is used to cushion the internal organs against damage, and cannot be used for energy. This is virtually the lower limit of body fat % that competition bodybuilders strive for on "game day".

If you are a semi-active individual, can still go to the gym, play recreational hockey, cycle, but are about 20 pounds heavier than you would like to be, your body fat % might be around 25%. Does that seem high? Don't forget that if your muscles aren't visible, they are covered by a thin fat layer, even though you might only look a little overweight "here and there". If you weigh 180 pounds, your LBW would be 75% x 180 = 135 pounds.

The "average" man's bodyweight is about 15% fat, and therefore his LBW is 85% of his scale weight The average woman's is about 25% and her LBW would therefore be about 75% of her scale weight. Discounting the fact that there is no such thing as an average man or woman, you could use those figures as guidelines if you are neither overly thin nor thick.

If you are quite overweight, can do very little walking or other activity without great exertion, float almost out of the water in a pool, you may have a body fat composition of 40% (or more). If you weigh 280, your LBW will be somewhere around 60% x 280 = 168 pounds.

You will have to guess-timate your body fat %, and hence determine your LBW, unless you have access to testing facilities, and many clubs DO provide this service. You will also have to determine your "Need Factor" from the following 5 choices, since your level of activity is also a determinant of your protein requirements.

Need Factor - NF - (general activity level)

0.5	Sedentary – no sports or training
0.6	Jogging or light fitness training
0.7	Sports participation or moderate training
0.8	Weight training or aerobic sports training daily
0.9	Heavy weight training daily
1.0	Double workouts daily – heavy load

Daily Protein Requirements

Now it's time to put it all together.

DAILY PROTEIN REQUIREMENTS (DPR)						
LBW (in pounds) X NF = DPR (in grams)						
LBW	0.5 NF	0.6 NF	0.7 NF	0.8 NF	0.9 NF	1.0 NF
90	45	54	63	72	81	90
100	50	60	70	80	90	100
110	55	66	77	88	99	110
120	60	72	84	86	108	120
130	65	78	91	104	117	130
140	70	84	98	112	126	140
150	75	90	105	120	135	150
160	80	96	112	128	144	160
170	85	102	119	136	153	170
180	90	108	126	144	162	180
190	95	114	133	152	171	190
200	100	120	140	160	180	200
210	105	126	147	168	189	210
220	110	132	154	175	198	220
230	115	138	161	184	207	230
240	120	144	168	192	216	240
250	125	150	175	200	225	250

An example of how to use the chart:

Let's assume that you are quite serious about increasing your muscle mass through some moderate weight training, and losing your excess fat through some light-medium aerobic work on alternate days. That puts you at an NF (need factor) of 0.8 Furthermore let's assume you are 190 pounds on the scale, but through critical self-appraisal using your mirror, decide that you are about 25% body fat, and that your LBW is therefore 75% x 190 = 142. On the chart above, where the 0.8 NF column meets the 140 LBW row, your daily protein requirement is 112 grams. These numbers are approximate, so don't get TOO uptight about adhering to them to the gram.

You need about 115 (to make the math easier) grams of protein, spread out over 5 meals, or roughly 23 grams each. Some meals will have more than others (for instance, your post-workout meal will be supplying protein for repair and growth, and hence will have a higher protein component than your smallish supper) but all meals should have some, in order to stay in positive nitrogen balance at all times. Refer back to Chapter 2 for more on positive nitrogen balance and its absolute necessity.

CHAPTER 7 Nth Degree Nutrition—
Food Combining

Back in Chapter 2, I stated that although the body needs certain nutritional elements, they are <u>NOT necessary at each meal</u>, which is our society's traditional approach to eating. It was also pointed out that, even if you don't wish to become a bodybuilder, they know a great deal about fat loss and muscle gain. The methods used by top champions embraces yet another concept, called Food Combining, which is a logical application of the chemistry and physiology of digestion, with special consideration given to the limitations of our digestive juices and enzymes.

Read two more pages of this chapter, and if it hasn't convinced you to read farther by then, just try to utilize all you can from the first six chapters, and skip forward to read Chapters 8 through 11.

The basis of this theory is as follows:

The Facts of Digestion

The nourishment our body receives is determined ONLY by the food we digest <u>properly</u> and assimilate into our bloodstream. Food which is not digested only wastes the body's energy as it passes through the alimentary canal. Bacteria in our intestines feed upon this undigested food, producing "rotting", and the byproducts of this are chemical compounds which are a real mess for our digestive tract to dispose of. This is a primary contributing factor in the causation of diseases, especially diverticulitis, colitis, and other itus's of the digestive tract.

Food combining is the sensible, logical way of consuming your foods so that everything stands the <u>best chance</u> of digesting properly. As bodybuilders, we strive to optimize all conditions that will promote muscle gain and fat loss – so it makes sense to consider a method of eating which makes digestion easier, is less complicated and more efficient.

The digestive system is a site of continual chemical activity that provides specific digestive enzymes required for the breakdown of different types of foods.

Starchy foods (concentrated complex carbohydrates) require an alkaline (basic) medium for digestion, which is supplied initially in the mouth by the digestive enzyme ptyaline. Protein foods require an acid medium for digestion, the enzyme pepsin and hydrochloric acid in the stomach. Those who have studied elementary chemistry know that acids and bases (alkalines) neutralize one another. Well, the same result happens when you eat a starch and a protein together. The digestive enzymes tend to neutralize one another, with the result that digestion can be impaired, or worse, stopped altogether.

The "Facts of Digestion" to remember are:

a) Either our food digests, or it doesn't.
b) We derive NO food value from undigested food.
c) Food, not digested, ROTS. As a result, it becomes the seed cause of almost all sickness – internal poisoning. It also produces bloating, gas (upper tract belching), and flatulence (lower tract methane emissions).

If you combine your foods correctly, controlling your weight will hardly ever be a problem; that bloated feeling will be gone; skin problems will disappear; constipation will be a thing of the past. You will be unlikely to become ill and you will start to achieve those goals, not only in bodybuilding, but in general overall health in a slimmer stronger body, that previously seemed unobtainable. The practical application of this theoretical knowledge has given us the "rules of food combining".

The Rules of Food Combining

1) Don't eat proteins and starches at the same meal. Recalling "the facts of digestion" there is no way this combination will

ever properly digest. What then, about meat and potatoes, meaty pizza, hotdogs? Take the hamburger, for example. It takes a series of acid digestive juices to digest the protein in the meat, and a series of alkaline digestive juices to digest the starch (bun). The juices cancel out one another somewhat (sometimes completely) and NO DIGESTION IS THE RESULT. This means: (horrors!) NO MUSCLE BUILDING MATERIAL AVAILABLE FOR GROWTH

It is recommended that if you do eat proteins and starches (rice, potatoes, pasta . . .) at the same meal, the meat or other protein part (fish, eggs, . . .) of the meal should come first, and the starch portion second. The protein goes to the lower part of the stomach (since it enters first) and digests, while the starch will digest in the upper part. Meals used to be prepared and served "in courses", which slowed the meal down and allowed for a more aesthetic appreciation of it. The individual servings would be small, and if presented in an order following the rules of food combining, would lead to better digestion as well.

Two different protein foods eaten together will rot in the stomach due to the widely differing character and composition. When we eat meat, for example, the highest concentration of hydrochloric acid is secreted within the first hour of digestion. When we ingest cheese, the highest concentration occurs in the third hour. Eggs receive the strongest secretion at a different time from either eggs or meat.

Therefore, do not eat eggs, meat, or dairy products at the same meal. Two types of flesh or two dairy products can be eaten together because they are similar in character and composition. Starches, by contrast, are not often as difficult to break down as protein, so more than one starch can be eaten at the same meal. For example, if you have pasta and lentils, or rice and beans at the same meal, they will be compatible in the stomach. Recall (or refer back to) in Chapter 2, we presented a chart showing how various carbohydrate sources (grains and legumes) could be combined to produce protein almost as high in quality as that from meat or eggs. It fits in perfectly with this first rule of food combining.

2) <u>Don't eat fruits with starches.</u> Starches are foods such as rice, potatoes and other "root" vegetables. The digestion of fruit requires hardly any time at all in the mouth and stomach, while starches require most of their time in these areas. If the fruit sugars are held up in the stomach while digestion of the starch continues, the fruit will ROT in no time. You will always have "problems" with this combination. The rule when eating fruit is:

EAT FRUIT AT A FRUIT MEAL

Another "fruit rule" is:

EAT MELONS ALONE OR LEAVE THEM ALONE

Melons combine with **NO** other food. They are already in their simplest form and require NO digestion time in the stomach at all. The stomach temperature is about 40 (degrees) C. Put a piece of melon in the sun at around 35C, and you can watch it rot before your eyes.

Although it's best to eat fruits and vegetables (the starchy ones, not the leafy, or salad ones) at separate meals, lemons and papayas are exceptions to this rule. Lemon juice can be used sparingly on steamed vegetables or salads, and papaya can be eaten with any kind of food. Papaya is the basis of many digestive enzyme tablets. And although tomatoes are (technically) fruits, they may be eaten with other vegetables.

3) <u>Don't eat fruit with protein.</u> The same reasoning applies here as for rule #2. If the sugars are held back in the stomach while the protein digests, you can count 100% on the fruit rotting, causing gas, bloating, and cramps (called "indigestion" quite rightly).

4) <u>Do not eat acidic fruits and sweet fruits together.</u> These two food groups definitely repel one another. There are <u>NO</u> exceptions to this rule. Acidic fruits have the juiciest fibers of all the fruits (oranges and other citrus types, apples, strawberries, grapes . . . .), whereas sweet fruits (dates, bananas, raisins, dried fruits . . . .) have no juice, are more concentrated, and take longer to digest.

5) <u>Do not mix more than 4-6 fruits or vegetables at a meal.</u> Remember:
The simpler the meal, the better you feel.

The preceding has been a fairly non-technical description of how various foods **should NOT** be combined. A few more facts should be explained if you wish to incorporate food combining into your nutritional plan for optimizing your physique and health goals.

Fats exert an inhibiting influence on the secretion of gastric juices, and this effect can last 2 hours or more. Because of this, protein foods that contain a large amount of fat, such as marbled or quite fatty meats, cheese, whole milk or nuts, will require more time to digest than proteins containing a lesser amount, such as the white meat of chicken or turkey, fish, low or non-fat dairy products.

When you eat a fat with a protein, its inhibiting effect upon the digestion can be offset somewhat by consuming an abundance of green vegetables (that are NOT considered starches), especially in their raw state.

Fats and oils are neutral (acidic/basic speaking) and although they retard digestion, they will <u>combine</u> well, and can be eaten with carbohydrates. Foods such as whole grain breads, and butter or avocado will combine well together (but will make you fatter).

It is recommended that you restrict fluids at meals. Too much fluid dilutes the digestive juices, making digestion that much more difficult. Don't "wash anything down"! If you do drink milk with a meal, keep in mind that it digests quite differently than the concentrated protein in meat, so this combination should be avoided. Have milk at other meals, with your milk and eggs protein shake for instance. Milk <u>can</u> be combined quite satisfactorily with starch, fruit or eggs.

Most of today's top bodybuilders eat many, SMALL, easily digested meals per day, as many as 6! Some meals may be all protein, others all fruit, others all complex carbs and starches. It is not necessary to eat several food types at one meal. By following the non-mixed meal plan you can still eat a balanced diet; you just do **NOT** eat all food types at each meal.

This is also a good way to prevent over-eating, as the body will only eat so much of one food at one sitting before it becomes distasteful. For example, how many eggs could you eat at one sitting before you lost your appetite for eggs? (NOTE: to keep your 1 meal protein intake less than 30 grams, 4 should be your limit). Or how many oranges? How many pieces of chicken? (OK, that one wasn't fair, especially if it was KFC, but you get the idea, right?) Eating only one or two types of food at each meal limits the amount of food eaten, but allows for maximum digestion, absorption and utilization.

When eating 4 or more meals per day, spaced at 3 to 4 hour intervals, it is to our advantage to have the stomach emptied of one meal before eating the next. It is easiest for the stomach to digest a single **concentrated** food at one time (called "mono" feedings). A properly combined mono meal will be out of the stomach in 3-4 hours.

The simpler the meal, the less complex the digestive process will be, and the more efficient will be the assimilation of nutrients from the food.

A meal should not consist of more than 4 or 5 foods. They must be eaten in chronological order, beginning with the easiest to digest first, to the more complex secondly, with the most CONCENTRATED last. An easy-to-remember "rule of thumb" on this is: eat the water-iest(?) food first, then proceed to each part of the meal that is less-so. It is important to remember that non-starchy vegetables (salads etc) are not concentrated foods, and can be eaten in combination with either of the concentrated food groupings (proteins or starches).

The following examples are listed in chronological eating order, beginning with the easiest to digest (water-iest), then to the most concentrated.

A) Mono-Starch Feeding: Raw vegetable salad
                         Beet greens
                         Broccoli
                         Brown rice (leaves stomach
                         in 3 hours)
B) Mono-Protein Feeding: Raw vegetable salad
                         Spinach
                         String beans
                         Fish (leaves stomach in 4 hours)

Red meat would take a little longer to clear the stomach, unless it is almost raw, which is great for those of you who prefer your steak rare.

While mono feedings are the simplest to prepare and clean up after, some people will still want to mix different <u>concentrated</u> foods at the same meal occasionally (i.e. have a steak and baked potato together). These meals will spend more time in the stomach and be more difficult to digest; therefore, when eating a mixed combination of 2 concentrated foods at a meal, you must eat them separately, and in proper sequence. We're getting back to the old "eating in courses" idea again. A meal consisting of a protein and a starch for example, must be consumed in the following order, for optimal digestion:

Raw vegetables
Green beans
Chicken
Yams

This mixture combination meal will leave the stomach in 4 to 6 hours.

PS Over the years I have read many articles extolling the theory, methods and merits of food combining. When I found one which explained it better than I could, it seemed only natural to use it. Why reinvent the wheel? Most of the information in this chapter was excerpted from an article by George Snyder. Having tried and been unable to locate him to request his permission to use it, I hereby acknowledge his authorship, with thanks. For readers who would like a more in-depth treatment of this subject, merely Google "Food Combining".

CHAPTER 8 How (actually) Do I Eat This Way?

In the preceding chapters, you have read about a lot of ideas that seem to make sense to you. They follow the old "eat your veggies and exercise" stuff that everyone has heard all of their lives, but it still may seem SO DIFFERENT from what you have been doing, possibly for years, that you can't imagine making such major changes in something so ingrained in your lifestyle as your eating habits. Everyone not only resists change, but almost fears it – because we are forced to go "outside our comfort zone" and actually learn and DO something new. And then, to have to make it habitual . . . .

No one likes to be told what to do – this statement is as true for 4 year olds as it is for me. They would rather <u>decide</u> what to do, and letting small children do this is (almost) never appropriate – they don't have enough experience to integrate their actions with the consequences of those actions. But adult readers of this manuscript have asked for sample eating plans and recipes; they have actually posed the question to me of this chapter's title. But . . . .

My experience through life so far has been that if I tell someone what to eat, and when, they will immediately start coming up with 101 reasons why they can't or won't. Back in the introduction, I stated that I would expect everyone to process the information presented, and then to question, analyze, experiment and think about how to personally apply it, because each of you is so different, not only in your parentage and upbringing, but in your age, weight, current level of fitness and health . . . . well, let's just say there are a lot of variables that make SPECIFIC suggestions almost useless. Even if you asked the question!

What **I will do** is to tell you how the results of **our** (my wife's and my) personal analysis, experimentation and label-reading have led to the contents of our pantry and refrigerator, when and what **we** eat, when and how **we** exercise, and put it all together in a lifestyle that still involves going to work, cleaning the house, seeing friends and relatives – you know, LIVING! You can then decide how to incorporate some or all of the changes **we** have made, into **your** lifestyle. What follows then, is what is keeping us fairly slim, strong and healthy even as we move through our sixth and seventh decades. The motto on the tee-shirts and tank tops I used to sell in my gym was "GET FIT – STAY FIT". We intend to stay that way! What about you?

Let's Stock the Pantry and Fridge

Fruits and Vegetables

We know that the only way we are going to eat fruit (for its Vitamin C, fiber, and simple natural carbohydrates) is if it is on hand and readily available. We buy several apples, bananas, peaches, strawberries, pears, apricots, a melon or two—whatever we like – and keep a few on a plate on our counter for a healthy snack anytime we want or to add to a packed lunch for work, and keep the rest in the fridge. We replenish this supply regularly, choosing a different one each time we have one, for the different nutrients they contain, letting none get soft (they decompose if not eaten).

We also know, for the same reason, that if we are going to eat vegetables (especially good for you if eaten raw) they must also be on hand. We regularly buy, cut up and keep in a large container in the fridge, broccoli, green peppers, turnip, carrots, celery, cauliflower, cucumbers – and anything else we can find that's in season or at least looks pretty fresh. We use the suggestions in Chapter 5 to make low-calorie dipping sauces and like them. Remember that the goodness is in the vegetable sticks, not the dipping sauce.

There should always be a salad in the fridge – a large bowl, more than a meals worth. If you are going to get out lettuce, tomatoes, mushrooms, bean sprouts, alfalfa sprouts, sliced almonds, cranberries – whatever you like – make a large enough quantity to last 2 or 3 days (without it starting to wilt and rot). Eat from it daily. When the bowl starts to get low or empty, there's one of tonight's jobs. Make another bowl full. Keep a shopping list on the counter at all times, and when any ingredient that you like and need runs out, replace it soon. Everything is always fresh and tastes the best that way. We buy or make only low-calorie dressings and use them sparingly. Again, the goodness is in the salad ingredients, not the dressing.

One of our favorite ways to have a protein meal is by combining a grain with a legume (see Chapter 2, the section on obtaining protein from non-meat sources) which completely gets around any cholesterol worries because what little fat there is, comes from carbohydrate sources. We fill our pantry with 540 mL cans (lots of them) of many different kinds of peas and beans (legumes) – black beans, red kidney beans, lentils, chick peas, navy beans, fava beans, Romano beans, soy beans, six bean blend . . . . and we get variety by opening a different one every couple of days. Each can will have between 7 and 15 grams of protein (read the labels). Open one of them, empty the contents into a strainer under a stream of cold water to rinse off the sodium it's packed in, and put it in a plastic storage container in the fridge. There's the legume part ready, enough for 2-4 meals, depending on how much protein **you** need in a meal. Next we always have lots of grains on hand, which can be brown rice, buckwheat, frozen corn (yes, corn is a grain), quinoa, barley, millet, whole wheat pasta (a form of wheat) . . . . We buy it in bulk (cheaper that way!) and keep lots of each in big glass containers in the pantry. We cook up a potful of any one of them, have some with our dinner, and store the rest in the fridge for future use. We always make up more than a meals worth when we're having dinner, so as to have enough on hand in the fridge to add to our legumes, and we vary which one is in the fridge at all times , again for variety.

Here's how to make a meatless protein meal then – follow "the two fist rule" from Chapter 6. Add equal quantities of legume and grain into a bowl (enough to make about two of your fists worth, or less), microwave it for a minute or so and consume it. You will be getting a few grams of protein from each ingredient, complex carbohydrates and fiber, some calcium and iron – a great pre-workout meal.

Nuts and Seeds

We buy one kilogram bags (bulk buying is always cheaper in the long run) of walnut pieces, whole almonds and pecans—and put half a cup of each in a smallish covered bowl on the counter. The big open bags left over we put in a large resealable bag and keep it in the freezer until the bowl gets empty. We often add a few cashews (unsalted if possible), raw unsalted sunflower seeds and raw pumpkin seeds to the mix. Remember that even though nuts are extremely fatty, at least the fatty acids are mono-unsaturated (MUFAs), so although nuts are (marginally) good for you, don't have more than a few at any given time. We sometimes sprinkle a few on our salad for a little treat. If your willpower is low, don't have them around at all until you get a grip on things, always remembering your goal of a slimmer stronger physique.

Dairy Products

We only buy skim milk now (mainly for making protein shakes), but used to buy 1% (fat) milk for many years. Since we drink one or two "shakes" each day, it makes sense to buy it in the most economical size, 4L at a time—providing you can consume it before it "goes off". No one needs the fat that homogenized (3.5% fat) and 2% (fat) milk contain, so try to cut down on them. We like cottage cheese (it can be used to make dips, too) and sour cream (can be used on baked potatoes) but only use the non-fat or 1% versions, using the same reasoning as above for milk.

This would probably be a good time to go back and reread Chapter 5 or I might end up repeating a lot of what's there. Reduce consumption of anything with a high fat content.

Now, Let's Eat!

First—calculate your lean body weight (LBW) as laid out back in Chapter 6 and FEED ONLY THAT. Use the need factor chart there and your estimated LBW to find how much protein you personally need at each of your 5 daily feedings.

Let's say that you have calculated that you need approximately 90 grams of protein daily, and know that this amount should be consumed over the course of each day in 5 meals – breakfast, mid-morning snack, lunch, mid-afternoon snack, and supper. Each meal should have at least 18-20 grams (5x18=90) of protein in it to stay in positive nitrogen balance, especially if it is a workout day. I like to get up early enough to have my workout (whether it's a gym day in the weight room, or an aerobics session) <u>before</u> my workday begins. After a good breakfast, I use the hour or so while that nutrition is beginning to digest, to answer emails, go through yesterday's mail, pay bills, or pack my mid-day meals if I will be out until suppertime. Then I exercise or walk, shower and get to work.

Between meal snacks are usually protein shakes, which can be made at the point of need if you are at home near all the ingredients, or blended up and taken with you to work in a small container. Here's how. Place a cup of skim milk in your blender, add a couple of spoonfuls of protein powder (read the label to see how much protein this will provide and judge accordingly), a couple of raw eggs, and a bit of banana or other fruit if you like your shakes flavored. Double the quantity if it will be 2 snacks for you later in the day. Mid-morning give it a shake and have half of it. Same in the afternoon. You will be getting 7 grams of protein from each egg, 9 grams from the milk, ? grams from the protein powder – more than 25 grams in total – great! If it's NOT a workout day, you can leave out one of the eggs because your needs are less. Too much protein is better than not enough; it just gets expensive if you overdo it.

Do you like <u>eating</u> eggs? Here's a good breakfast, and a low-calorie way to make it. Add (only) a teaspoon of olive oil to a small frying pan, set to medium heat. Spread the oil around and crack in 2 eggs. Add a little water, no more than a ¼ cup, and cover the pan with a lid. Stay close by – it won't take them long to be lightly poached. Use the time to toast a piece of whole wheat bread. With this method, you use less oil than with normal frying, and you don't lose so much of the egg's white as in normal poaching. Have a cup of skim milk with it. Notice that no mention was made of bacon with it – it's TOO FATTY. So what do we have? – 7 grams of protein from each egg, 4 grams from the piece of toast, and 9 grams from the cup of milk. 27 grams! If dry toast doesn't appeal to you, try spreading a thin layer of ripe avocado on it– there is a little bit of fat there, but it comes from MUFAs (mono-unsaturated fatty acids—the good kind found in nuts and olive oil) rather than from the saturated fats that come from butter or margarine. Our early meal should be robust enough to fuel the morning's activities.

Lunch, whether we're at home or away at work, is usually something left over from a previous supper. We always cook more at suppertime than we can consume at that meal, for this very reason. It might be a small fillet or 2 of fish, a lean hamburg patty, a piece of liver, a couple of pieces of chicken, some whole wheat pasta. If you have had steamed broccoli, green beans or cauliflower with your meal or . . . . , any that was left over can go into your lunch too. Many people will have access to a microwave oven at work, so you can warm it up a bit – I like it cold just as well. Have a baggie full of the cut up vegetables from your tray in the fridge to have with it, and a couple of pieces of fruit for anytime during the day that you start getting the munchies. If there are no nutritious leftovers sometime, open a can of water-packed tuna, rinse off the sodium in your strainer, add a small spoonful of mayonnaise and a little diced raw onion. Mush it all up the way you like it. Put it in a plastic container, along with a fork and a piece of whole wheat bread, and voila! 30 grams of protein from the tuna, and from the slice of bread—complex carbs and 4 grams of protein. You could take 1/2 the mixture if you don't need that much protein, saving the other ½ for another time. Do you like sardines? A single can of water-packed sardines has 17 grams of protein. Check out the protein, fat and carbohydrate content of your favorite lunch foods and decide which ones to eat and which to avoid on that basis. You can calculate the protein in your lunch if you wish, but the main thing to keep in mind at all times is the fat content of everything passing between your lips. Remember your goal at all times. Gravy is NOT a beverage!

Another breakfast or lunch suggestion is a combination of whatever grain and legume you currently have in the fridge. Warm it up at home or at work (take a spoon or fork along!) and you have a quick one-dish (easy cleanup) meal. You can constantly vary the combinations to find which ones you like best, and if you want a bit more flavor, try stirring in a spoonful of Worcestershire sauce, soy sauce, steak sauce, ketchup, light ranch dressing, mustard . . . . after you've put it into the container you are taking to work. You will be getting some protein (the combination will be just as good for you as if it came from a meat source), lots of complex carbs for slow energy release, fiber, blood sugar control, as well as some vitamins and iron.

You may have noticed that no mention has been made anywhere in all this about desserts. We might have ice cream once or twice **a year**, if someone is having a birthday. We don't ever follow nutritious meals with high-calorie, nutrient-less pies, cakes or any other kind of baked goods. We <u>never</u> have candy, chocolate, doughnuts or cookies in the house. Butter tarts are about the only exception, and that is only around Christmastime. You can simply say "no thank you" to hostesses or restaurant employees when desserts are offered. If you have been careful about what you've already consumed in terms of quantity (the two fist rule) and fat content, you certainly won't be hungry, even if it looks tempting. ALWAYS remember your goals.

Supper should always be smallish, because your caloric needs are almost nil during the evening and during sleep. Remember and review the section called The Metabolic Needs Curve back in Chapter 6. Unless you have your weights workout late in the day after work, your supper can have a lower protein component than the other meals, but if your schedule makes late afternoon workouts necessary, you will need to replenish your system according to the information in Chapter 6. Having a bowl of salad before your smallish supper and keeping any evening snacking to low fat sources and small quantities will make for a more restful sleep. You need <u>at least</u> 8 hours. Personally, I find that fitting 1 to 1 ½ hours of health-building activity **daily** into an otherwise crowded life is only possible if it's done <u>early in the day</u>. It energizes me at work, the eating schedule proposed keeps me alert (at least more so than if I don't pay attention to it!), and by going to bed early because I am tired after attending to all the other necessary daily duties, I tend not to waste time that I used to. Mowing lawns in the summer, shoveling snow in the winter . . . . should all be seen as more exercise and part of an active lifestyle, not drudgery. Playing with children and grandchildren is **at least as important** as watching fictional TV characters, playing video games, or spending time poring over Facebook or U-Tube videos for hours. Going to bed early enough to get all-important recuperation and rest makes arising early enough to train easier, and somehow it seems to be less intrusive on my other daytime activities. You may find that working out after work in the afternoon is best for you, and sometimes it's true for me as well, but the main point I'm trying to constantly hammer home here, is that "I don't have time to do all this" is NOT TRUE! You do have time – you just need to get rid of whatever former habits were keeping you from being slimmer, stronger, healthier and happier.

"Changing You" may turn out to be more than just about your physique or your body's fat percentage. It may lead you into a deeper analysis of your priorities in life, who you hang out with, what you do in your "free time", the types of things you read, the places you would like to see . . . .

CHAPTER 9 Aerobic vs Anaerobic Conditioning

When I first opened The Change Room gymnasium, I bought not only free weights, exercise benches, and machines, but I also purchased 2 step-up machines and 2 exercise bicycles. These 4 pieces of equipment were for warming up on, prior to using the weights, but some of my customers liked to get on them and stay on them for lengthy periods of time. This type of training is called "aerobic" training. You use a lot of air (oxygen) doing aerobic activity, and it can be running, spinning, rowing on an ergometer, using an elliptical machine, stair-climbing, fast walking or jogging on a treadmill or outdoors . . . . anything that gets your heart rate elevated and keeps it there for a sustained length of time. Conversely, anaerobic activity (weight training) involves very little movement and is not performed in a continuous manner. You may get a little short-winded near the end of a heavy set, but you recuperate very quickly, and then do it again.

These two types of training balance each other beautifully, for the benefits of one complement the other, and you can do them on alternate days. Muscles primarily derive their fuel from the breakdown of glycogen (blood glucose) in the cells during anaerobic activity (not in the presence of much oxygen). The energy needed during aerobic activity (you're sucking in all the oxygen you can for prolonged periods) comes primarily from the oxidation of fatty acids. This is truly where fat reduction kicks into high gear!!

Close to the beginning of Chapter 3, it was suggested that people who want to lose some weight and "tone up" should not only incorporate some or all of the nutritional suggestions in this book (50% of the process), but start getting into a regular exercise regimen (the other 50%). Three short workouts (of less than 1 hour) per week with weights, and a walking program on alternate days is a good place to start. Then take a day off for other enjoyable activities with family and friends. The hardest part of the process is wrapping your mind around the whole idea, and then BEGINNING. The next hardest part is STAYING WITH IT week after week, for months and months!! The great part about it is that you will learn to love it, and you will get positive feedback (results) almost immediately. Start slowly, but don't quit – not ever. Once you can walk steadily for an hour, you needn't take longer – you are ready for light aerobics.

Here's what aerobics will do for you.

1) increases fat metabolism
2) increases your basal metabolic rate (your "idle" speed)
3) decreases your blood pressure
4) decreases your resting pulse (your heart gets stronger)
5) decreases your cholesterol (the "bad" LDL kind)
6) increases your cholesterol (the "good" HDL kind)
7) increases circulatory efficiency
8) you have better workout recovery

Hmmm – it almost sounds like a valuable thing to do!! Here's how.

Target Heart Rate Calculations

To achieve the above effects, learn how to measure your resting pulse. Take it each morning, as soon as possible before doing anything active. You will need a watch with a sweep-second hand; count your heart beats on the inside of your wrist, or at the large artery on your neck for 15 seconds, then multiply the result by 4 to get your "basal" or resting heart rate in beats per minute. Write it down in a notebook. When it starts dropping, you'll know the aerobic effects are beginning to happen. You will also need to calculate what's called your "target heart range".

Calculate your target heart range as follows:

Formula: 220 – age = maximum heart rate

65% to 85% of maximum heart rate is the target zone

(220-age) X 65% = lower heart rate limit
(220-age) X 85% = upper heart rate limit

Sources vary widely on how long an aerobic workout is best, but you'll soon know what's right for you. Each session should last at least 15 to 30 minutes, and some people like to do a lot more, up to an hour. Don't worry if you can't get your heart rate high enough at first, or if you CAN, but can't keep it there long enough. Just as with the original walking program when you progressed from "ground 0" to walking for an hour, then walked steadily faster until you could cover much more ground in the same amount of time, keep track of what you do during each aerobic session. You may have to do the initial sessions at less than the lower heart rate you've calculated, but keep it there for at least 15 minutes. Steadily force yourself to work harder until you are "in the target zone", and pretty soon you won't have to keep taking your pulse to know when you are there. It's a feeling that's accompanied by a certain rhythm of motion, a certain level of respirations (breathing heavily, but still able to speak), and probably some sweating. Once you can get into the target heart rate zone, each session stay at it for a few minutes longer. By then, you'll fit right in with all the other nuts who wish to have a healthy middle and old age.

Procedure

1) warm up 5-10 minutes
2) spend 20-40 minutes in your target zone, monitoring your pulse
3) warm down 5-10 minutes (to slowly reduce systemic adrenaline)

Frequency

Do your aerobic training 3 times per week minimum, to get a sustained metabolic effect and improvement in blood lipids (lower cholesterol).
Alternate aerobics with your resistance work (free weights and/ or machines).
The metabolic effects can last 15-24 hours (sources really vary on this, too).

Sessions done early in the day burn more fat than those in the afternoon.

Additional Exercise Information (you're really getting into it now!)

Let's have a deeper look at the two broad categories of exercise, aerobic and anaerobic, and see how they relate to losing or gaining weight. Remember the person who pointed at his protruding belly and said "I just want to get rid of this!"? He needs to learn that it is impossible to spot reduce any area of the body through exercise or by any other means. Exercising any body part results in an increased metabolic rate throughout the body, and fatty acids will be mobilized from fat stored throughout the body, not selectively at the area worked.

The term aerobic means to utilize oxygen and aerobic exercise increases the body's oxygen uptake, causing you to breathe harder and more frequently. The extra oxygen is used to burn fuel for muscular energy. That fuel can be either glucose (stored as glycogen) or fatty acids (stored as fat) or both. These two fuels undergo processes which change them into ATP (adenosine triphosphate, for you biochemists).

ATP is a compound that stores energy in its molecular bonds until required by the body to perform work. ATP is what the cells use to power muscle contraction, for the active transport of nutrients across cell membranes, synthesis of body compounds, and secretion of hormones.

Exercising at low to moderate levels of intensity, up to about 60% of maximum effort, allows the body to use both its glycogen and fat reserves, with mostly fat supplying the energy. These fuels are converted into ATP in the presence of oxygen; they are metabolized aerobically.

When exercise intensity exceeds 60% of maximum effort, the muscles cannot get oxygen fast enough. The body cannot produce ATP from fatty acids without oxygen. However, glucose **can be** converted into ATP without oxygen; it can be metabolized anaerobically.

Aerobic metabolism produces 36 molecules of ATP from each one of glucose, plus up to 131 molecules of ATP from each fatty acid molecule oxidized, **once that process gets started.** Anaerobic metabolism (bodybuilding with weights, shot putting, powerlifting etc.) produces only 2 molecules of ATP from each molecule of glucose. That's why you can't exercise really intensely for very long without fatigue.

Some glucose is changed into lactic acid as a byproduct of anaerobic metabolism. The buildup of lactic acid is what causes that burning sensation in muscles that have been worked hard, and inhibits the mobilization of free fatty acids from the fat stores. Your body burns less fat and uses mostly carbs for energy and that is why you must have lots of carbs before a weights workout, and sip on a maltodextrin (complex carbs) drink before and during it. Later, when oxygen returns to adequate levels, most of the lactic acid is changed back into glucose.

Here's the exciting part if you wish to lose fat!

The process by which fatty acids are mobilized, or released, from fat storage is slow to get started. Therefore, at the onset of aerobic exercise, most of the fuel is glucose. **Only after 10 to 30 minutes, depending on the individual, does most of the energy come from fats.** I believe that this is what accounts for what is often called "getting your second wind"—extra energy from a totally different source kicks in!! The longer the aerobic activity is performed, the greater will be the percentage of fat mobilized for fuel. Long-distance runners are usually pretty fat free – this is why!

Anaerobic exercise, contrary to popular belief, does promote reduction of fat deposits, although not as fast as aerobic exercise. Indeed, no exercise is completely aerobic or completely anaerobic. Even during high intensity effort, some fuel is metabolized aerobically, but as I've stressed so many times previously, the bottom line in terms of weight reduction is to burn more calories than you take in.

Aerobic exercise, because of its stimulating effect on the heart and lungs, tends to increase the efficiency of the cardiovascular and respiratory systems. Your heart (which is a muscle) gets stronger. By increasing the volume of blood pumped with each beat, the number of beats per minute decreases. That's why I suggested earlier, that you get into the habit of checking your resting pulse rate first thing in the morning, preferably even before you get out of bed. When it starts to decrease, you know your heart and lungs are becoming stronger and more efficient (the aerobic effect). Regular endurance (aerobic) exercise can lower the resting pulse by 20 beats or more, but must be performed at least 3 times per week, and preferably more often. The "at least" part means that if you reserve one day per week to do "other things", that on some workout days you would do BOTH a weights workout and an aerobic session, or on some days you could do 2 aerobic workouts, preferably, but not necessarily, separated by several hours. Each aerobic session should last at least 15-30 minutes, but highly motivated individuals can do more. That's you, right?

Exercising with weights and machines is valuable for shaping, toning and strengthening the muscles of the body. As it is usually performed with moderate to heavy resistance, this type of exercise is mostly anaerobic, being brief and intense. It can have an aerobic effect with the use of lighter resistance and using higher repetitions, and this is usually referred to as circuit training, a totally different way of using weights. See Chapter 11 for some very basic sample routines.

An important prerequisite to building muscle with weight exercises is a high level of the male sex hormone testosterone. Young men have more than older men, and so have an easier time building muscle in the gym. Women have relatively low levels of testosterone in their systems, and therefore should not worry about developing large unfeminine muscles with free weight and machine exercises. A woman can, however, develop a strong, shapely athletic body with this type of program.

Well, are you going to go "all the way"?? Here's how. You are going to get so focused on your goal of being fitter, healthier, better looking physically (with or without clothes on), more energetic—that you will spend 1-1 ½ hours per day *doing something*, every day, devoted to a **changed you**. You will train at home or in a gym <u>every</u> day – alternating bodybuilding exercises and the aerobic activity you most prefer. You can mix the aerobics part up, varying the activity from one session to the next if you have access to different types of equipment. All of them are safe, low impact (they don't jar your knees and ankles), they are convenient, non-weather related and your progress is easy to monitor. A partner who shares the same goals really helps, for you encourage one another during temporary motivational lapses.

CHAPTER 10 Gymnasium Training Principles

Knowledge is Necessary

The change process is not a "maybe" proposition. The body will always adapt to changed conditions (i.e. starve it and it gets smaller). The starvation diet would be the "changed conditions" and the size reduction would be the body's adaptation.

Consider the biceps muscle. Suppose you want to change the height of its peak when flexed. You are going to need as much knowledge, and understanding, of that muscle as possible, to change its shape. You will need to know how it works, where its attachments are, and the various exercises that can be used to help change its shape. Only then will you be able to "work" it in a specific way to induce a specific adaptation—in this case, a higher "peak".

You cannot know too much about the science of bodybuilding and the workings of the human body. You must gradually learn how the muscles of the body work to produce motion of the various limbs, and how they work together to provide locomotion for the body as a whole. Most people think they know this information intuitively, but that often turns out not to be the case. Often when I'm teaching someone how to do "lat pulldowns" and I say, "contract your lats as you pull down on the bar", they are unable to do so at first, because they have never experienced the feeling of deliberately contracting a muscle, nor do they know where the lat muscles are. This ongoing learning process is aided by reading in the fields of physiology and anatomy. The popular fitness magazines such as "Men's Fitness" and "Muscle and Fitness" contain many interesting articles each month, by experts in these fields, as well as training articles by professional bodybuilders. Take in all you can, to help maximize your results.

Weight Selection

Especially during the first few workouts, novice trainers have an almost uncontrollable urge to go all out for a maximum lift. This approach is not only incorrect, it can be extremely harmful. You can hurt yourself <u>badly</u> doing this. The prime requisite is that the exercise be done correctly, to achieve the desired effect.

Weight training for physique building is not just a matter of lifting a weight from point A to point B. The idea is to <u>use</u> that weight, <u>as a tool</u>, to stimulate muscle growth in a previously identified area. Since the weight must be moved through a very specific pathway, proper exercise performance is absolutely essential and you must use weights light enough to perform the movements perfectly.

You should spend from 5-15 minutes at the beginning of each workout doing light stretching movements, to reduce the chance of hurting yourself before you've "warmed up". Do some neck rotations, shoulder shrugs, arm circles, trunk rotations, and deep knee bends – all without weights – before beginning your routine, until you feel quite limber. You could jump on an exercise bike for 10 minutes to help get your system warmed up and ready. Use this time to think about your last workout, and to identify any areas that may be hurt, as opposed to just being a little tight or stiff. You should work lightly through general stiffness, but avoid further stressing a sprain, a strain, or a torn muscle. Leave them alone, working around them if possible, but this will be extremely infrequent if you learn and practice proper exercise performance from the outset.

All new exercises should be done with medium-light weights for the first 5-10 workouts to minimize tissue damage or injury, and to prevent excessive soreness the following day. Later of course, it will be your definite goal to stress (this does not mean to injure!) your muscle tissues to the maximum, so that, in the presence of great nutrients coursing through your bloodstream, they will repair themselves "and then some". They seem to get used to the fact that this might happen again (and it will, 100's of times over the years ahead), getting bigger and stronger to handle the anticipated workload increases. Regular breaking down of muscle cells is the name of the game, but it must be done with control and a well-thought-out program for achieving specific results.

Workout Tempo

The unsuccessful bodybuilder often thinks nothing of resting up to ten minutes between sets, talking to friends or reading a muscle magazine. I see it all the time and these same people often are unaware that more than a minute or two has elapsed. There should never be more than three minutes between even the heaviest sets, sometimes as little as 30 seconds. The main consideration here is that your heart rate gets back to "about normal" and your breathing stabilizes somewhat, before beginning another set. You should be able to speak normally, but don't <u>do</u> much of it.

Taking longer between sets than it takes to change plates or dumbbells, and to record the poundage used in the previous set, will cause you to lose not only your "pump", but also your overall energy level. To make real progress there must not only be a regular cadence (or rhythm) to the repetitions during your set, but the rest periods between sets must also be very regimented. Your muscles will thrive on this discipline. Proper workout tempo results from a positive attitude and a complete singleness of purpose. Certainly, you will not seriously challenge your potential to its limit by training in an undisciplined manner. Maintain concentration, not only <u>during</u> a set of a particular exercise, but also during the metered rest period. Keep fired up and "zeroed in" for maximum results.

Breathing

While nothing is more instinctive and natural than breathing, during heavy exercise sets it seems to become less so. Many times I'm asked "How should I breathe during this exercise?" The rule of thumb on this question is: **Breathe out with effort**.

Never try to breathe in and out through the nose only, when training vigorously. The nose is too small to accommodate huge air (oxygen) intake volumes, so open your mouth and gulp it in. Your muscles need plenty of oxygen, so make sure they get it.

Many men and women inhale deeply before doing an abdominal "crunch" and then hold their breath throughout the contraction. This is incorrect. Do <u>not</u> hold your breath. Following the "breathe out with effort" rule <u>means</u>: there must be as little air in the lungs as possible as you exhale completely and contract the abdominal muscles.

There's no rule about one breath in and one breath out PER REPETITION. Take an extra breath or 2 whenever you need to.

Exercise Selection and Order

At the beginning of your training, the whole body gets exercised in each workout. If the weights selected have been light enough, there should be little or no soreness "the morning after". If there is, then during your next workout (usually 2 days later), repeat the exercise that caused that particular muscle to ache, as before, but use less weight. In full-body workouts, each major muscle group should be exercised with specific exercises, and you gradually become aware of exactly which part of a muscle that the exercise "hits".

In general, the larger muscles should be worked before the smaller ones, so the order you follow will be: THIGHS – BACK – CHEST – SHOULDERS – TRICEPS – BICEPS – FOREARMS – CALVES – ABDOMINALS. You will do 2 or 3 exercises for each area, one "set" of each, during your first few workouts. Your main job at the beginning of your training will be to learn how do these basic exercises in perfect form, while steadily raising the weights you can handle. The control you must develop in these early workouts provides the basis for unlimited future development, and, as in most human endeavors, poor habits learned early are usually hard to break later. In this sport, poor exercise habits will lead to zero progress and recurring injuries.

Remember from chapter one that there is NO SUCH THING as spot reduction. The whole body must be exercised, because fat loss is "systemic", not "spot specific". Since your ultimate goal is perfect proportion, you must resist the temptation to work your favorite or most developed body parts to the exclusion of the weaker areas. Sub-par body parts must, if anything, be given extra attention to bring them up to the level of the rest of your body, and then increase all muscle groups together.

As your training progresses and you go from being a novice to an "intermediate", to an "advanced" trainer, you will undoubtedly begin using a "split" system of training.

This method of training involves dividing the major parts being exercised into two or three separate workouts, allowing you to exercise each part more intensely, while at the same time allowing more recuperation time for rebuilding your muscles. Even in split routines, larger parts should be worked before smaller parts, since your energy level is greatest at the beginning of a workout, and can be devoted to muscles requiring large input.

Workout Length and Recuperation Time

Each workout should last no longer than one and a half hours. At the beginning 1 hour will be more than enough! If your workout takes longer than this, you are either doing too many sets, or taking too long between them. The energy from your pre-workout meal (1-2 hours before) will be running very low around the end of a 2 hour workout. Workouts of this length will suffer from lack of intensity and gains will cease. It would be better to have two shorter, but more intense workouts per day than one three hour marathon session, but this method is best reserved for pre-competition bodybuilders. This type of training is professional, and is called "double-splitting".

Each workout should be followed by complete relaxation, for at least several hours. In the beginning, a novice can train as often as his or her enthusiasm will allow, providing adequate recuperation is taking place. Keep in mind that muscles don't grow and become stronger in the gym. The "hypertrophy" (or growing process) occurs between workouts. The micro-trauma and cellular breakdown that we induce through heavy training must be repaired, and the muscles rebuild themselves larger and stronger to prevent more damage. We will continually place ever-increasing demands on them, and they will constantly strengthen to meet these demands. This is called "**progressive resistance** training" – **we always strive to increase the weight handled or the repetitions performed with the same weight at each workout**. Obviously, if the muscles haven't recuperated completely, they cannot be expected to grow stronger.

Overtraining

When we train too hard, or too often, or for too long, a situation arises called "overtraining". The result is a LOSS of muscle tissue, hormone depletion and weakness. Ironically, a person suffering from this overwork and staleness often looks as though he hasn't been doing <u>enough</u> work, because of the stringy and smoothed-out appearance of the muscles. The symptoms of overtraining are: loss of appetite, irritability, insomnia, nagging injuries that won't go away, no gains. Some experts say that there is no such thing as overtraining, just under nutrition and lack of recuperation time.

Personally, I think it's usually a combination of all three. In bodybuilding, we are always "on the edge". We want to train hard enough to induce muscular growth, but also we must ensure enough recuperation time to prevent overtraining. And our nutritional intake has to be very closely monitored. It's a fine line to have to walk, but <u>you will learn how</u>, easily. Learn to listen to your body's responses. Scientists call it biofeedback.

Gym Etiquette

Perfect exercise performance to me means one other thing as well. Although on the last rep or two of your heaviest sets, an audible grunt may escape your lips from time to time, you should try never to do this, <u>deliberately</u>. Every gym has one or two people who groan, moan, or even scream during (supposedly) heavy work. They are doing it <u>for effect</u>, and think that people around them will be impressed. Nothing could be further from the truth. Truly powerful people don't "show off" in any way, certainly not audibly, preferring to conserve the energy used for groaning and using it for making their muscles contract during yet another repetition.

Furthermore, you should never do anything in the gym that will distract someone else's concentration. Don't talk to people <u>during</u> their set. Wait until they set the weight down. Don't disturb their rhythm or concentration. Don't walk between them and a mirror they may be facing.

Respecting one another is a great universal goal and most people practice it unconsciously (I like to think), but some people seem to forget that this rule for getting along socially, applies equally well in the gym as elsewhere. Each person in the gym is striving to change something about themselves, both mentally and physically – and keeping this constantly in mind should be "the great equalizer".

The trainer with three years experience and very noticeable development has <u>NO</u> rights greater than those of a novice. He doesn't have the right to monopolize the squat rack, or the lat machine, nor does anyone else. If anything, more experienced gym members should "bend over backwards" to <u>help new people</u>, remembering how unfamiliar and nerve-wracking this whole process can be, especially at the beginning.

Help each other through heavy lifts. "Spotting" is a technique that requires careful learning, and you'll be glad when someone you've shown how, gives you a perfect "assist".

Always put your plates and dumbbells away after use. Not only will this practice help reduce tripping accidents, but it's only polite. Why should anyone have to remove four 45 pound plates from your bar before they do their shrugs with 60 pounds?

Since everyone needs a short break between sets, it makes sense to share benches and machines, especially if the gym is a little crowded. It takes very little time to change plates, if that is necessary, and both people can act as encouraging support spotters for one another. It's also a good way to get to know other members. Remember, we're all in this together.

We all want changes!

There are many advanced training techniques that are definitely beyond the scope of this book. There are ways to break "plateaus" or "sticking points", as well as methods for increasing workout intensity. You will learn these methods by reading muscle magazines, or from the manager of the gym you attend. By then, you will be very knowledgeable indeed, will be changing your routines instinctively when necessary, and will be well on the way to achieving your goals. Good luck!

Chapter 11 Novice and Intermediate Workouts

There will be a little overlap between the general principles stated in Chapter 10 and this one. I've added this short chapter, because many people have told me "well, that all sounds pretty straight forward, but I still don't know what to **actually DO**".

First, I'm going to tell you a VERY short story.

Once upon a time, a long long time ago, in a distant galaxy far far away (OK I'm not sure about that last part!) there was a young man who lived on a cattle ranch. His parents fed him very well, and he was quite husky from all the hard work that was always required. He had seen a strongman act at the county fair the previous year, and felt that he could do that kind of thing too, if only he could get even bigger and stronger than he already was, and one night in bed, he came up with a plan to accomplish exactly that.

It was calving season at the ranch, and he knew he could easily pick up a new born calf, since they generally weigh less than 100 pounds when born. His idea was that in addition to all his other daily jobs, he would pick up that calf every day as it grew, and that as it gained weight, his muscles would have to get stronger and stronger, to enable him to keep it up all summer. From previous years, he knew that the calf would end up being around 600 pounds in the fall, so that by then he should have the strength of Hercules. Mid-way through June our young hero's dream was dashed on the rocks of reality. Although he did increase his strength somewhat at the beginning, the increasing resistance that the calf was daily providing exceeded his ability to adapt, and there soon came a day when he could no longer pick it up. At first, he thought it was because it was all squirmy and hard to get his arms around, and that may be true in part, because there are men who CAN pick up 600 pounds (if it's on a barbell), but they didn't get that strong in a six month period. His plan turned out to be just too ambitious, and the point of the story is that although you will start slowly, your strength absolutely has an upper limit, especially over short time periods like 6 months or a year. Try to enjoy the time you spend on your new-found sport. It's much more than a pastime – it's health in action! And it is one of the few sports that you can do for the rest of your life.

If you have already had some training experience, you can probably just skim through these final few pages. You certainly do not need the expense of hiring a personal trainer. For the rest of my readers, the first time you enter a gym can be pretty intimidating. Some gyms have the look of a medieval torture chamber; more modern ones may resemble a space ship, full of gleaming electronic equipment with flashing LED display monitors. At first you won't know what some of the equipment is for, and everyone else will seem to know SO MUCH MORE than you do . . . .but ALL OF THEM started out (at some point) at exactly your stage. Realize that they are **all** there for the same reasons you are – they want changes, and still do – and in general they will be friendly and helpful. In a few months, you will undoubtedly see someone walk in with a nervous look on their face. It's their first time and you may remember then how YOU felt originally, not like "the old pro" that you will become! But that's for much later.

At present, I am going to assume that you are indeed a true novice, and are taking your very first workouts as a result of reading this book. There will be a bit of a steep learning curve ahead of you yet, in addition to applying the nutritional advice given previously. Even if you have some previous experience using weights, but have been away from it for quite a while, you should treat the first dozen or so workouts as having three functions and three ONLY. They are:

1) Learning how to DO each exercise in perfect form.
2) Finding out the weight that you can comfortably handle in each exercise without causing undo soreness the next day.
3) Adopting a method of record keeping that will ensure continual progress.

I will explain how to do all of these.

Learning Proper Exercise Form

Unless you know me personally and can come to my home gym for some hands-on training advice, you will need to find a training partner who already knows the basic exercises and how to perform them correctly, or to join a gym where someone will "walk you through" the following programs for a few weeks until you are comfortable and more confident. The exercises that I propose you begin with will be well-known to anyone there, and you should easily be able to get some free advice. There are two aspects of using weights for strengthening muscles that you must always keep in mind.

1) Use full range of motion

Muscles are attached by tendons to the bones on either side of a joint, and when they <u>contract</u>, one of your limbs moves. There is always a different muscle on the other side of the same joint that has to <u>extend</u> to allow that contraction. To move the limb back to its starting point, the second muscle contracts while the first one extends. Let me give an example. Hold a book in your hand with your arm straight down by your thigh. If you contract your bicep muscle, which is attached below your elbow joint by a tendon and up by your shoulder at the upper end, the muscle will "pull" your forearm upwards until the book is at your shoulder. If you deliberately stop the motion before the book is all the way up, you have not used the "full range of motion" of your bicep, and hence it has not been completely exercised. While your arm is in motion upwards, the tricep muscle on the back of your arm needs to extend. To lower the book to its starting position, the contracted bicep relaxes (extends) while the tricep muscle contracts.

Whenever a single joint moves, pairs of muscles are always involved, and it is our goal to strengthen these muscles through specific exercises, very gently at first until you understand what and why you are doing them. If you are pressing dumbbells overhead from a starting position at your shoulders (to strengthen the deltoids), press them ALL the way up. Don't short-change the benefits you want by shortening the full range of motion possible.

If you are doing deep knee bends, go ALL the way down – the knee joint (unless it is injured) is meant to be flexible enough to allow the full squat position and once again, stopping short is a bad habit to get into – you compromise future performance. Later on, when using weights in this exercise, you should stop your downward movement in squats when your thighs are about parallel to the floor, to prevent excess knee strain.

2) Use NO extraneous body motion (called "cheating")

Another habit often seen in novice trainers is the tendency to load the bar up with more weight than can be easily handled, and then by bringing into play almost their whole body they use momentum to raise the weight, swinging it up and down. An example would be holding a barbell in front of the body preparatory to doing barbell curls for the biceps, then bending forward at the waist and heaving it up to the shoulders using the momentum created by moving the hips rapidly forward. This is called "cheating", not as in a card game, but as in cheating yourself of the benefits that come from using strictly controlled form. In all likelihood the biceps might not be involved in the movement AT ALL! The person is getting the barbell up to where it is supposed to get, but not by exercising their biceps, plus there's a good chance of straining one's lower back doing this. It would be much better to decrease the weight on the bar to an easily manageable amount that will enable you to do many repetitions with a regular cadence, and through the full range of motion. Now, how much weight is enough?

Finding Your Starting Exercise Poundages

I've read many books by champions addressing this issue, and it seems that they have forgotten their humble origins. One was saying if you can bench press 315 pounds easily, just add 25 pounds to each side of the bar, and carry on until that becomes easy, then do it again. Wow – I've trained for 30 years and have never been able to bench 315. But the theory is correct – you do have to start **somewhere** and work your way up, but I don't suggest using 315 pounds.

When it comes to novice trainers, there sometimes is <u>no amount</u> that is light enough. I had one young woman starting out, and I showed her how to do supported (you hold on to something) deep knee bends as part of the warm-up procedure. She barely could do 3 or 4, and was immediately almost injured. We went on to do some upper body exercises with 5 pound weights, and within 30 minutes, she had had enough. The next day she phoned me to tell me that she could barely get onto or off the toilet, because her legs ached so terribly. We had to progress VERY slowly, and that's all right. Better to begin with <u>no</u> weights and work up slowly, than to let ALL of one's muscles atrophy like that. She later told me that the last actual exercise of any kind that she had done was playing volleyball in high school 10 years earlier. I am certainly not criticizing her, but her example served to show me that the starting level for anyone should never be determined by "how they look".

So – what to do? I cannot give you a certain starting poundage for any given exercise. For each exercise on the workout lists that follow, you will have to pick up some small dumbbells (never mind what people around you are using – this is NOT a competition) and try to do the exercise for the suggested number of reps (repetitions). If they feel **really** light when you first pick them up, rerack them and pick up the next heaviest set. You will soon learn that just because you can <u>pick up</u> a weight does not necessarily mean that you can perform a certain exercise with it in proper form. If the weight you selected feels quite light, go through the motions anyway, and use the time to learn what constitutes perfect form and full range of motion. If it truly felt like you had a bag of marshmallows in each hand, do not record the poundage used—immediately do it again with heavier dumbbells. You will have many more workouts to adjust what you should be starting with. If you have picked up a weight that felt good, but once on a bench attempting to use it realize that it is too heavy right away, immediately get up carefully, put it back on the rack, and start again with something lighter. This procedure won't take long. Within 3 workouts you will know what weight you should be handling, whether the exercise calls for the use of dumbbells, a barbell or a machine that lets you control the weight used with what's called a pin stack. With these machines you insert a pin in a stack of plates and try to do the exercise. If you "pinned in" too much, you will immediately know it. My suggestion in all cases is to use the lightest weights available or the minimum number of plates on a stack-type machine, and work your way up.

Especially for the first few workouts, resist the temptation to really push yourself. Even after a pretty mild-feeling effort, you may be a little stiff the next morning, because your muscles are being challenged to do something they have **never** done before. If there is no residual soreness, great! – you didn't overdo it, and you will have plenty of time to increase the loads you handle. If you **are** a bit sore, perhaps only in one or two muscle groups, make a mental note of them and during your next workout, decrease the weights you used in the exercises designed to affect those areas. Make sure you strive for perfect form with no cheating motions, through a full range of motion. You have a day off before you go back to the gym and tomorrow you should feel less stiff. Go for a walk, or some other easy aerobic activity to flush nutrients into and through your muscles – they need to rid themselves of waste products (mainly a buildup of lactic acid from over-exercising causes muscle soreness), and after another good sleep, you should be ready to go back in for your second workout.

You are going to go into the gym 3 times per week for the next few months, and during the first month, it's all about learning the exercises and hopefully enjoying yourself. If you are careful in applying the suggestions mentioned above, you should never be very sore or stiff, and you certainly should not incur ANY injuries. Each exercise is designed to work a certain muscle or muscle group, through a very specific pathway, to induce a specific response – an increase in strength. You must pay attention to how you feel during each repetition, controlling the movement – doing this creates what experienced trainers call the "mind to muscle link" – your body learns exactly how it is supposed to do the exercise, and if you lose your balance or your concentration during a movement, that is usually when a small muscle pull might creep in. It happens occasionally, so try to "get into that neural pathway" to avoid strains.

In progressive resistance weight training we NEVER go for all-out maximum lift totals, nor do we do endless sets of very high repetition work. Our goal is to strengthen our muscles so that everyday life becomes easier and more enjoyable, and to build a bit of extra muscle. Why? So that we can burn off any excess fat we may be carrying <u>in them</u> when we do our aerobic training on the alternate days. At the beginning, you will find that you can use heavier weights almost every workout, and you might start thinking like our friend earlier who dreamt of soon being able to pick up a full grown cow. What you **are** going to need is a small notebook to keep track of what you actually do during each workout, knowing full well that the early apparent strength gains **will** slow down. You must not be discouraged by this, because a lot of those quick gains in poundages handled are due to the strengthening of your tendons (which is good!). Remember that muscles themselves grow relatively slowly: here's how to keep track of it.

Record Keeping

Keep records of the weights you use and the number of repetitions performed <u>in perfect style</u>. This habit places less reliance on your memory, and since you should be constantly striving to increase either the weight you use (even just 5 pounds) or the number of repetitions (even **one more** than during your last workout) you perform, your record of your last workout will serve as a performance level to be exceeded. Without records, it is all too easy to use the same or lower weights than previously, and this practice will only lead to physique maintenance or deterioration, not improvement.

The Range Method

Especially in the first weeks of your gym work, you should try to raise the weight you handle in any given exercise every 4 or 5 workouts and I believe that the best way to accomplish this is through the use of what I call "the range method". It works like this. Suppose you are going to do a set of 10 repetitions of dumbbell bench presses. Let's assume for the sake of the example that you can handle 15 pound dumbbells and can get through your whole set without losing proper form. Good. Sit up, stand up and rack the dumbbells. Go immediately to your notebook and write down 15X10, to indicate that you used 15 pound dumbbells, and that you did 10 repetitions in good form. You will move from exercise to exercise, and after each one you will make a similar notation as to what exercise you did, what weight you handled, and how many repetitions you did. After your workout, probably less than an hour if you are not taking too much time between sets, head off for a meal or other activity that you need to do. When you next "hit the gym", when you come to do your dumbbell bench presses, look at your notebook, and see that you did 10 reps last time. With the previous performance as a challenge to be exceeded, this time do 11 reps, and providing that you can do them all in good form, write down 15X11, and repeat this procedure for all your other exercises. Next workout, go for 12 repetitions – say to yourself, I did 11 last time, surely I can do one more than that, then do it, and write down 15X12. After another workout, you can probably write down 15X13. This will then be 4 workouts at 15 pounds for that exercise, and if you feel you could do more, then during your next workout, start with 20 pound dumbbells, but only do 10 repetitions, writing down 20X10. Do you see how this pattern will find you writing down 20X13 three workouts later?, at which time you can raise the weight to 25 pound dumbbells, decrease the repetitions again, writing down 25X10. Each workout using the range of repetitions of 10,11,12,13 requires that you are progressively doing a little more "volume" of work each workout, and when you hit the upper end of the range, you raise the weight being used. Because it is heavier than before, don't expect to be able to do as many repetitions – drop back down to 10—the bottom end of "the range". It still counts as progress because you are now using a heavier weight. In the novice workouts which follow, if the suggested reps start at 12, the range method will take you through 12 13 14 15 before you raise the weight handled, and if it says start with 8 reps, the range method will take you through 8 9 10 11 before you raise the weight.

Two different scenarios may arise. You may find that although you can do 15X11 for a certain exercise, that during the next workout, you can still only do 15X11, or perhaps only 15X10. You may "fail" at 10 or 11, meaning that either you cannot perform the 12th rep, or that if you do the strain is too great, and you lose proper form, or cannot go through the whole range of motion you were attempting. This could be the result of a poor sleep, not paying strict enough attention to your food intake or its timing, mental stress from some source (your concentration is off), you have a cold, lots of things. Don't worry about it. Merely write down how many repetitions you DID do in proper form, and next workout try to exceed it. This program you are on won't necessarily be a steady linear progression, always upward – you know that you will never be able to lift that cow, so be content with any small gains you can make, and if you hit a "plateau" for a workout or two, so be it.

The other situation that often arises, especially in the beginning, is that of wanting to do too much. Even if your muscles aren't overly stiff or sore the next day (and I hope they aren't – you might quit!) resist the tendency to do 20 repetitions during a set. If the weight is so light that you can do more than 10-13, it is too light to begin with. Quickly find weights that enable you to do the required amounts of repetitions. At the end of each set, you should be just able to finish it, or perhaps feeling that you could have done another 1 or 2. There shouldn't be too much gas left in your tank, but even if there is, just increase the reps by one. There are so many workouts ahead that you don't want to stall out in the first month due to over exuberance, or by having picked up an injury.

You may find that some muscle or muscle group responds better than others to the exercises. The weights you can handle or the repetitions you can perform just keep going up – you start liking those body parts and often people tend to exercise them even more because they respond so well. Try to resist this tendency – your goal is, if anything, to bring lagging muscle groups UP to your favorites, striving for balance and symmetry. Other muscles will seem to stubbornly resist your efforts after a while, but don't avoid them – they obviously need extra attention

– try rearranging the order in which you do your workout, putting the slow responding muscle group first in your workout, while your energy is at its highest. If, after a few more workouts you are still discouraged, it is usually time to change the exercise(s) you are doing for that body part, and there are lots of choices. Ask the gym manager for suggestions, or any other knowledgeable trainer. Just be sure not to add exercises to an existing program or your workout will become too long. Never make it drudgery. There are many ways of breaking these "sticking points", which you will learn as you stay with your training. I have found that the best way to stay interested is to have a training partner who has roughly the same goals as you do. You commit to each other to always be there at workout time, help "spot" for one another during heavy sets, and coach each other when style seems to be going off. You can't always tell about that if you train alone. The other huge advantage that good training partners bring to one another is that the chance of both of you "being down" and wanting to skip a workout on the same day is quite unlikely. If one of you is wavering, the other one says "c'mon – you'll be glad once we've done it!" Against your will you go along with him or her, and an hour later, you are energized, refreshed, and truly thankful to them for helping keep you true to your goals.

Sample Workouts

I am going to suggest exercises that can all be done with dumbbells, because all gyms have a full selection of them. Later on, as you progress and learn from others, you will move on to using barbells and (probably) machines, such as a lat pulldown machine for your back, leg extension bench, hamstring curl bench, or cable apparatus for the smaller muscle groups such as triceps. Using the principle of working the largest muscle groups first, the order will be: Thighs–Back-Chest-Shoulders(deltoids)-Arms(biceps and triceps)-Abdominals. I am leaving out calves and forearms for now – you can add them in later if you wish, but for now just realize that every time you pick up anything you are using your wrists and forearms, and that during each step that you take your bodyweight is momentarily lifted with the calf of one leg.

1) Novice Workout

Warm up your joints and muscles by doing light stretching for a few minutes. Reread the "Weight Selection" section of Chapter 10 regarding warm-up procedures, and follow the suggestions there before every workout.

Thighs – Lunges (holding dumbbells)
Back – One-arm dumbbell rows
Chest – Flat bench dumbbell bench press
Shoulders (Delts) – Alternate overhead dumbbell press
Biceps – Alternate dumbbell curls
Triceps – Kneeling dumbbell kickbacks
Abdominals – Crunches – use no weight, start with 10 and work your way up to 30 or so

For each exercise, do a set with a weight that will allow 12 repetitions, rest a minute or two (not more!), then pick up a slightly heavier weight and go for 10 repetitions. The first set should be fairly easy, and serves as a warm-up for the second set. The second set will be a little harder because you have raised the weight, but you don't have to do as many repetitions.
Move through the list above, doing 2 sets of each, remembering to write down what weight you handled and how many reps.
You will have done 14 sets in all, and in well under 1 hour.

Two days later, go through the same procedure, referring to your notebook to see how many repetitions you will try for according to the range method described above.

You can do this workout for 2 or 3 weeks, going in to the gym 3 times per week, always with at least one day between for recuperation, and on those days "off" you can be following the walking program described in Chapter 4.

When you feel that you are ready for **more volume** of exercise, you should add a third set of each exercise. As above, the first set will be well within your ability to complete and serves as a warm-up for the second. Both of them serve as a warm-up for the third set, which should feel like real effort. Maintain proper style and control. You will again pick up a heavier weight than in the second set, but you will start with only 8 repetitions.

When deciding how much weight to use in each set, try to make the jump between set 1 and 2 larger than the jump between set 2 and 3. For instance, if you are using 10 pound dumbbells for your first set, try to use 20s for the second (a jump of 10 pounds), but only 25s for the third (a jump of 5 pounds). Always stay within your ability to use proper form for the required number of repetitions.

At this point you will now be doing 21 sets – 7 exercises, 3 sets of each, and your workout still shouldn't be taking much more than an hour, if that. If it is taking more time than that, you are resting too long between sets. It never takes more than a long minute to do 12 repetitions of anything. Take a minute or so to relax a little, record what you did, and keep going. 3 minutes per set X 21 sets = about an hour.

2) Intermediate Workout

You can stay with the above workout for as long as you wish, providing you aren't getting bored, and you are still getting gains, as measured in your notebook by increasing weights handled and repetitions performed. Never change a workout as long as you are progressing. The time will come, however, when you want more variety and that can only be achieved by adding extra exercises for each muscle part, but we don't want the time spent in the gym to increase. Therefore it will be necessary to split your workout into two separate ones, and do them alternately, but you will not be training the whole body in each workout as with the novice workout above. I will call them Workout "A" and Workout "B", and you will have to alter your record keeping system a little – you will need two pages instead of one. If you regularly work out on Monday, Wednesday and Friday each week, this next system will have you doing Workout "A" on Monday and Friday the first week, and Wednesday the second week. Workout "B" will be done on Wednesday the first week, and Monday and Friday the second week. Alternating the 2 different workouts gives more intensive work and variety to each muscle group while allowing maximum recuperation time for the body parts being worked, while still getting 3 workouts per week.

As above with the novice workout, always start with some stretching and joint articulation movements such as neck rotations, arm circles, trunk rotations, supported deep knee bends. You can do your abdominal work (crunches) at the beginning if you wish. They are a great warm-up for everything that follows in your workout.

By now, you know your way around the gym, have probably made some new friends, and have seen them doing exercises on equipment you haven't tried yet. Now's the time!

Workout "A"

Thighs – Leg extensions (special bench) – 3 sets 12-10-8
      – Lunges (holding dumbbells) – 3 sets 10-8-6
Chest – Flat bench flyes – 3 sets 12-10-8
      – Flat bench dumbbell bench press – 3 sets 10-8-6
Biceps – Dumbbell concentration curls – 2 sets 12-10
      – E-Z curls (curved grip barbell) – 2 sets 8-6
Abdominals – 2 sets 20-30 (make them "burn")

18 sets, less than 1 hour

Workout "B"

Back – One-arm dumbbell rows – 3 sets 12-10-8
      – Lat pulldowns (special apparatus) – 3 sets 10-8-6
Delts – Dumbbell lateral raises – 3 sets 12-10-8
      – Alternate overhead dumbbell presses—3 sets 10-8-6
Triceps – Triceps pushdowns – cable machine – 2 sets 12-10
      – Seated alternate dumbbell French press – 2 sets 8-6
Abdominals – 2 sets 20-30 (make them hurt!)

18 sets, less than 1 hour

For all exercises you will use the "add-weight" system as you go through the 2 or 3 required sets, adding weight on each set but attempting fewer repetitions because of this.

In both workouts, make sure you try for 1 extra repetition per set, per exercise, each workout using the range method. You will always get the feeling of having progressed that way, and it's true, even if you don't "go up" in <u>every</u> exercise <u>every</u> workout. The smallest progress per workout should be found gratifying enough to keep you coming back for more in the weeks and months ahead. You can stay on these beginner programs for 4-6 months.

There are 2 ways you can use the 2 workouts.

Alternate them Monday, Wednesday, Friday, and take 2 days off. The off days needn't be Saturday and Sunday. If you work at your job Monday to Friday, you might wish to have one of your workouts on the weekend and your 2 day "break" during the week when your free time is less available.
The other way (especially if you are really enjoying your gym time) is to do workout A and B on consecutive days, take one day off, then the 2 workouts again consecutively, then 2 days off. You are now getting 4 workouts in the week instead of 3.

You now have enough information to start with, and if your gym isn't very helpful in answering questions, feel free to email me at the address at the back of this book – **<u>your</u>** progress toward **<u>your</u>** goal is my greatest hope for you, and you are going to be a wonderful example to SO MANY others!! I truly wish you great success.

CONCLUSION

In the winter of 1989-1990, I wrote a weekly column in the local newspaper entitled "Changing You". I was trying to promote the concepts that I taught at "The Change Room" gym, and those 12 columns formed the basis of the original form of this book. I didn't know, really, if anyone read them or not – I got so little feedback. My friends made the odd positive comment, if I prodded them, but it was interesting writing to an unknown audience nevertheless. I allowed myself the daydream that I was a lonely voice calling out in the wilderness, trying to spread the fitness message where fitness consciousness had barely reared its head.

I extolled the virtues of exercise; how it lowers your resting heart rate (making it last longer); how it lowers your blood pressure and "perceived" stress levels; how it cures poor posture and all its attendant aches and pains. I explained how, by reversing the muscle-loss/fat-gain spiral with bodybuilding exercises and attention to proper nutrition, **we can cure obesity** and stave off some of the effects of aging. I maintained that building a fit muscular body increases <u>any person's</u> self-confidence, and that a healthy strong body is the proper outward manifestation of a mind that is fully alive.

Our bodies are meant to be flexible, agile and powerful right through to old age, not wracked with preventable diseases caused by terrible eating habits and lack of exercise. In issue #9 of my short column-writing career, I pointed out that the twentieth century "discovery" of exercise was nothing new genetically. Our glandular and hormonal systems were programmed for a life of action and a diet of natural food (probably eaten one type at a time as it was obtained – early food combining?) thousands of years ago. Aside from obesity, which is usually a factor in these others, five of our society's most destructive ailments – heart attack, stroke, cirrhosis of the liver, diabetes, and atherosclerosis (hardening of the arteries) – are nutrition related and in large part due to inactivity. I maintained that <u>only the individual</u> is responsible for his own well-being. No one else can make you well – YOU have to take charge of <u>your own</u> wellness. Why not let the "normal" diseases of middle and old age pass you by? I asked.

Fast forward 21 years to the rewrite of, and additions to "Changing You". Not surprisingly, I've managed to get 21 years older as well, yet still carefully watch my diet, exercise with weights 3 times per week, and do aerobic work 3-5 times per week. Writing now as a 63 year old man, I'm no longer surprised to be able to quote from <u>last week's</u> newspaper the following "new" health news:

Health News – 9 reasons to exercise. Looking for some motivation to leave the computer, TV, or dining room table? Here are a handful of reasons.

1) <u>Stroke:</u> Aerobic exercise lowers the risk of stroke. In one study, women who walked at least an hour a day had a 40% lower risk than those who walked less than an hour a week.
2) <u>Heart Disease:</u> Aerobic exercise cuts the risk of heart attack by 20-35% in most studies. Women walking briskly for at least 30 minutes per day, 5 days per week, had a 30-40% lower risk of heart attack or other cardiovascular event than sedentary women.
3) <u>Broken Bones:</u> Weight bearing aerobic and strength training exercise 3-5 days per week can increase – or slow the decrease in—the density of spine and hip bones.
4) <u>Diabetes:</u> Moderately active people have a 30-40% lower risk of type 2 diabetes than inactive people. Normal weight women who were sedentary had twice the risk of diabetes, and obese women who were sedentary had 16 times the risk, compared to normal-weight active women.
5) <u>Depression:</u> Active people are 15-25% less likely to be diagnosed with depression than inactive people. In people with depression, moderate-to-vigorous aerobic exercise (30 minute 3 times per week) decreases symptoms.
6) <u>Blood Pressure:</u> Forty minutes of moderate-to-vigorous aerobic exercise 3-5 times a week lowers systolic blood pressure by 2-5 points. That may not sound like much, but it would save thousands of lives per year.

7) Mitochondria: Aerobic exercise increases the size, number and activity of mitochondria, the fuel burning centers of your muscle cells. Mitochondria don't function as well in people who are older, obese, or diabetic.
8) Arthritis: If you have arthritis, moderate-intensity, low impact exercise for 20-60 minutes 3-5 times per week can reduce pain and disability. Both aerobic and muscle strengthening help.
9) Falls: Older adults who are physically active have about a 30% lower risk of falls. The activity includes moderate-intensity strength training for 30 minutes 3 times a week, and walking for 30 minutes at least twice a week.

So – we've come full circle. The topics covered in this book weren't even new when I was on the rowing team in university. I practiced them in a youthfully haphazard way for 20 years, then opened a gym, learned a lot more, and produced the original version of this book. Twenty more years have passed; the information has been revised and expanded to suit a more enlightened, questing group of people, and it is my great hope that many will take it to heart, and then put it into practice as a lifestyle of activity, supported by sound nutritional principles. Teach it to your children. Model it for your grandchildren.

If you have read this far, and value it, please don't LOAN your book to someone else. Suggest they buy a copy from me. Keep yours as a reference book, and refer to it every once in a while, to keep you on track toward your goal of a slimmer, stronger body.

Yours in health and fitness,
Cole Clifford

PS To order copies for your friends, family and fellow fitness buffs, or with questions about the content and ideas within "Changing You", please feel free to email me at:

cclifford@lakescom.net

CPSIA information can be obtained at www.ICGtesting.com
Printed in the USA
LVOW082034121012

302516LV00002B/1/P